Baking Technology and Nutrition

Baking Technology and Nutrition

Towards a Healthier World

Stanley P. Cauvain and Rosie H. Clark
BakeTran
Witney

WILEY

This edition first published 2019

Registered Office(s)
John Wiley & Sons, Inc., 111 River Street, Hoboken, NJ 07030, USA

Editorial Office
The Atrium, Southern Gate, Chichester, West Sussex, PO19 8SQ, UK

For details of our global editorial offices, customer services, and more information about Wiley products visit us at www.wiley.com.

Wiley also publishes its books in a variety of electronic formats and by print-on-demand. Some content that appears in standard print versions of this book may not be available in other formats.

Library of Congress Cataloging-in-Publication Data

Names: Cauvain, Stanley P., author. | Clark, Rosie H., 1966– author.
Title: Baking technology and nutrition : towards a healthier world / Stanley P. Cauvain, Rosie H. Clark.
Description: First edition. | Hoboken, NJ : Wiley, [2019] | Includes bibliographical references and index. |
Identifiers: LCCN 2019017437 (print) | LCCN 2019021606 (ebook) | ISBN 9781119387121 (Adobe PDF) | ISBN 9781119387169 (ePub) | ISBN 9781119387152 (hardcover)
Subjects: LCSH: Baked products. | Baking. | Nutrition.
Classification: LCC TX552.15 (ebook) | LCC TX552.15 .C385 2019 (print) | DDC 664/.752–dc23
LC record available at https://lccn.loc.gov/2019017437

Cover Design: Wiley
Cover Image: © karp5/Shutterstock

Set in 10/12pt Warnock by SPi Global, Pondicherry, India

10 9 8 7 6 5 4 3 2 1

Contents

Preface

There is no doubt that we are living at a time of global food crises; food depravation and malnutrition continue, for various reasons, to blight some parts of the world while elsewhere consumer obesity has become a major issue. Bakery food products have a significant role to play in both scenarios because of the ubiquitous nature of baked products manufacture. In the case of potential malnutrition, the fortification of wheat flour can make major contributions to improving health. In the case of the obesity epidemic, there is the potential for bakery foods to contribute to nutritional enhancement and health through reformulation to increase fibre, reduce energy density, salt, sugar, and fat. In setting out to write this book we recognised the dual role that the development of healthier bakery food products could play, as a response by bakers to government-led initiatives (fortification) and interventions (reformulation), and from consumers seeking healthier lifestyles (consumer-pull).

The manufacture of bakery products involves changes of state (e.g. dough to bread) which are the result of complex interactions between ingredients, recipe, and processing. The different sub-groups of bakery products are delivered through the management of these complex interactions This means that changes in one aspect in the different bakery product relationships has significant 'knock-on' effects for the processing requirements and final product quality. Such complexities are not always immediately recognised when potential dietary changes are only recommended or implemented from a nutritional viewpoint. Even when nutritionists and bakery technologists work closely together, the product development road is a long and often arduous one.

In writing this book we have considered the potential for the nutritional enhancement of baked products from a number of different viewpoints. We have attempted to enlighten nutritionists as to the complexities of baking and bakery product quality and, at the same time, present to bakers the opportunities that new 'healthier' bakery products could bring to their businesses. In identifying the latter, we have illustrated a few of the possible paths for the development of new products, some traditional and some less so.

Ultimately the success or otherwise, of nutritionally enhanced bakery products in the market place lies with consumers. There will be huge differences in attitude between consumers requiring improved basic nutrition and those fortunate enough to live in parts of the world with largely unrestricted food sources. For the latter group of consumers, the abundance and variety of bakery products available, results in greater emphasis being placed on the sensory pleasure associated with the eating of the products, rather than the needs for basic nutrition. Within the fortunate consumer groups the challenges for improving the nutritional background of bakery foods are greater for bakers. However, many bakers are cognisant of their potential contribution to reducing the global obesity crisis and its related health issues, and will no doubt continue to make positive efforts to meet nutritional targets. We hope that in some way this book will help them meet the challenges of developing those healthier bakery products.

Stanley P. Cauvain
Rosie H. Clark

1

An Introduction to the History of the Manufacture of Bakery Products and Relevant Studies in Human Nutrition

1.1 The Historical Development of Bakery Products

Bakery products as we know them today, have a wide range of forms and commonly, the most important ingredient in the recipe is wheat flour. It is probably about 20 000 years ago that humankind discovered the nutritional qualities of the wild grass progenitors of modern wheats in the Middle East (Ucko and Dimbleby 1969). Recent research has shown that the processing of grains, the manufacture of dough and baking of bread, extends back to around 15 000 years ago (Arranz-Otaegui et al. 2018) pre-dating the arrival of 'agriculture' by some 4000 years. Thus, it appears that so-called 'hunter-gatherer' peoples, were the first to turn grains into a palatable and easily transported (convenience) food. Early breads were almost certainly similar to the flatbreads which are still available in the Middle East and many other parts of the world, today. This basic form of (unleavened) bread became the first processed and convenience food. No doubt it was not long before these early bakers discovered that the addition of salt improved the flavour profile of the mixture. Leaving the uncooked mixture exposed to the atmosphere would make it susceptible to contamination with wild yeasts and it would not be long before people began to appreciate the improvement in digestibility that would come from a spontaneously fermented mixture, and the light and aerated bread that came with it; a process still practised today and commonly referred to as 'sour dough' or artisan breads (Figure 1.1).

Baking Technology and Nutrition: Towards a Healthier World, First Edition.
Stanley P. Cauvain and Rosie H. Clark.

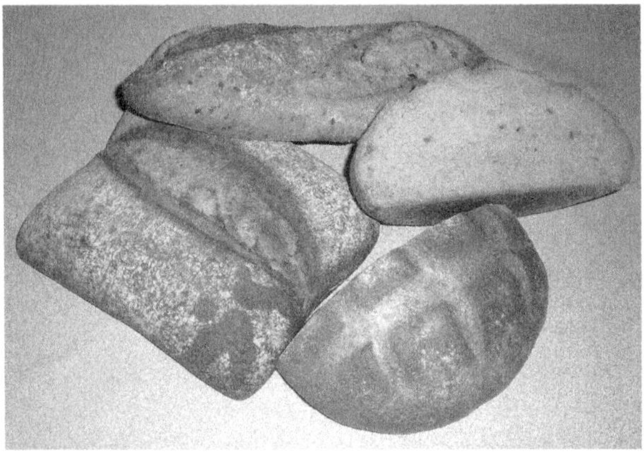

Figure 1.1 Sour dough and artisan breads.

From these early beginnings, producers of bread began to establish the principles which still underpin breadmaking today; mainly the manipulation and control of fermentation which delivers the carbon dioxide gas allowing the dough to rise and yield a light, aerated structure in the final product. Gradually from the early stages of domestic production, the baking of bread and other grain based products, moved to becoming a specialised craft and in civilisations like those of ancient Egypt, it developed into an industrialised form (Ashton 1904). The techniques recorded by the Egyptians in the paintings adorning the walls of a number of tombs, include the kneading of the dough in large tubs and the oven baking of the mixture in a mould are – the origins of the modern pan bread production. At this time, sifted wheat flour would have been chosen by the rich, while lower classes and workers would have had to make do with much coarser bread, often based on a mixture of wheat and barley (Bailey 1975).

Bread quickly became established as a staple food, classically referred to as 'the staff of life', because of the plentiful supply of wheat and other grains. Very soon those skilled in the art of baking began to add other ingredients to improve flavour and nutrition, and introduce new forms and shapes. Even in ancient times, fat was added to the dough to improve the softness and mouthfeel of the baked product, and honey to provide sweetness, yielding products which are referred to in ancient texts as 'cakes'. Such products were often associated with festivals and baked in moulds of various forms, often to represent animals, and in ancient Greece occasionally more erotic forms (Toussaint-Samat 1992).

By Roman times, baking had become a skilled art and a wide variety of products were available. At this time, the milling of wheat still mostly consisted of producing a coarse wholemeal flour. Following traditions established in ancient Egypt, this coarse wholemeal flour was sieved to remove a proportion of the bran, with the remaining flour being used for products to feed the elite classes. At the highest levels in Roman society the flour used would be comparable to the white flours of today, although with a little more bran than we are used to. These white flours were particularly favoured in the production of sweetened forms of breads and included confections based on 'flaky' pastry sheets, with cheese and honey figuring in the recipes. Even in Roman times, the position of bread in society was more than just providing sustenance, as exemplified from the quote from a satirical poet, Juvenal, in the late first century CE about satisfying the common people with bread and circuses; given the violent nature of the latter, this represents a curious juxtaposition of sensory pleasures. The ever-increasing need of the Roman Empire to provide its population with basic foods, was a key driver behind the conquest of the grain rich growing regions of France (known then as Gaul) and Britain. This was to introduce the Romans to very different forms of wheat, in particular spelt, the flour from which was used to make a very round and soft off-white loaf in the Gaulish regions. Today there has been a resurgence of interest in ancient grains in relationship to their potential contribution to 'healthy' eating, as will be discussed below.

Bakery products have a long association with symbolism and rituals and this resulted in the development of products that we would still recognise today, many of which are still associated with the festivals of many religions. In the northern hemisphere, there has been a long tradition of making special breads to celebrate successful harvest of wheat, for example the traditional wheatsheaf and representations of the Cornucopia (horn of plenty); the latter stretching back several thousand years. Not all traditional products are associated with religions, for example the croissant is believed to have been invented by the bakers of Vienna to celebrate their timely warning against the attack by the Ottoman Turks in the fifteenth century. There can be more mundane reasons for creating special products or marking the surface of bread with symbols. For example, bread produced for the Roman legions was stamped with the relevant legion number to ensure that the product reached the relevant customer. The origins of cutting the dough's surface to create a particular pattern, has the pragmatic function of differentiating your product from that of another baker; such practices still exist today but have often become enshrined in the desirable characteristics of the product, for example the London Bloomer illustrated in Figure 1.2.

As far back as the time of the Egyptian Pharos, baking had become a large-scale state sponsored and organised industry in order to feed the large workforce necessary for construction of monuments like the pyramids (Samuel 1999). While the individual bakeries were small in size, the organisation of the production was based on creating central sites to deliver the mass of bread required. The Romans were to employ a similar approach to feeding their armies throughout their empire. Other examples of centralised or state organised bread production, include those associated with the sites of major castles and monasteries, some of which could have had resident populations equivalent to small medieval towns, and certainly larger than villages. In medieval towns there would be many bakeries but of a less organised nature, however, the continuing rise in bread production in the medieval period was to lead to the voluntary organisation of baking in the form of guilds and other similar organisations. In part this was a response to regulatory pressures from local and regional authorities to ensure that consumers would be getting the required quality of

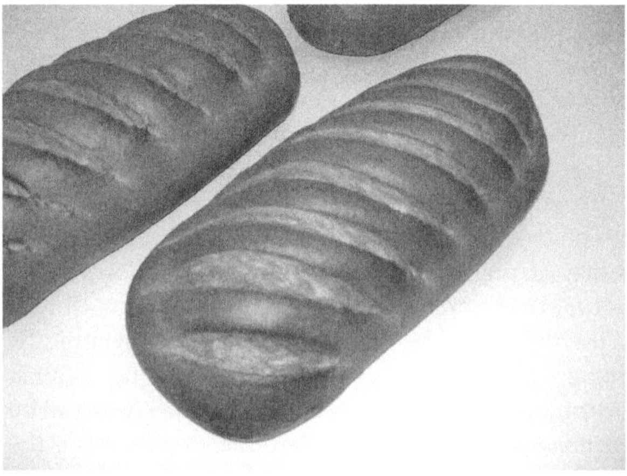

Figure 1.2 London (UK) bloomer loaf.

product, at appropriate prices. Crucially in medieval periods, significant measures were undertaken to control the weight of bread at the point of sale (Bailey 1975) and in many cases the price was set by governments. In the modern era, legislative control of bread price is less common, though control of bread weights is universally applied and there may be a maximum limit to product moisture or minimum solids control to ensure that consumers get what they pay for.

Alongside bread, other forms of bakery products were evolving, so that by 1440 there are references to pastry cooks, and the baking of cakes and biscuits. There were pies in both savoury and sweet forms using flaky and filo-style pastries. Around the same time, there are references to fritters, wafers, waffles, and tarts. The growing appetite of the western world for sugar, known from ancient Roman and Greek times through the access to the 'Sakcharon' (sweet reed) and based on raw materials from the Indian sub-continent, was accelerated by the voyages of discovery to the Caribbean, and it became a key ingredient of many baked products and other confections. The high price of sugar at this time would have restricted its consumption to the higher social orders, with those of lower class having a diet in which bread still played a critical role. The inability of some states to provide sufficient bread could have serious consequences, even leading to rioting. An illustration of how important bakery products had become by the seventeenth century is the (in)famous quote from Marie Antoinette who, on being told that French peasants were rioting because they had no bread, is supposed to have said, 'Let them eat cake' (the traditional translation of the French phrase 'Qu'ils mangent de la brioche'). Though this attribution is unproven, it has become a long-standing illustration of the importance of bread in society and of the divide between the elite and the common populous. If the French peasantry lacked bread, they were most unlikely to have access to sweetened bakery products.

Gradually, the artisanal base of baking was to give way to increasing industrialisation as the Industrial Revolution gathered pace in eighteenth century Europe. With increasing access to reliable sources of power, mills and bakeries were able to grow in size and provide large-scale production of bread for the industrial workers of the developing cities. At the same time, the knowledge of the world around us was expanding as a result of the work of scientists. In the context of baking an important discovery came from the work of Louis Pasteur on fermentation. His studies on yeast fermentation were to eventually lead to the manufacture of modern bakers' yeasts (Cauvain 2015). With a reliable source of carbon dioxide production, bakers were able to produce more consistent products. Around the same time, the large wheat growing areas of North America were being developed and the importation of the strong wheats that they yielded, changed the quality of the flour that millers could make available to bakers. On the back of such events, there was a general shift towards the consumption of white bread throughout all communities; white bread was no longer the province of the elite.

The association between the consumption of white bread and a rise in social standing has a long history (Bailey 1975; Marchant et al. 2008). Even in relatively modern times this phenomenon has been observed. For example, before 1990 large-scale production of bread in South Africa was focussed on a high extraction rate flour (~80% of the grain) which was used to deliver a standardised loaf controlled by the government of the day. When deregulation arrived in South Africa, there was an immediate shift by the populous to the consumption of white bread. This choice of white bread as a primary product is still being seen today with the increase of bread consumption in communities throughout South East Asia. While the products may have some historical links with bread production in Europe, the bread recipe in South East Asia is quite different and typically contains high levels of sugar and fat. Indeed, without sugar many South East Asian consumers will refer to the bread as having a 'sour' taste, even though sour dough technology has not been used for its production. The consumption of bakery products is now so widespread that they have become an integral part of consumer choice, even in countries that cannot grow wheat. There is no doubt that part of the reason for such developments is related to delivering sensory pleasure – taste, flavour and texture – and convenience. With their convenient forms and good shelf-life bakery products are often seen as readily available alternatives to more traditional diets; for example, bread needs no preparation in order to provide a satisfactory breakfast meal, even if it has to be toasted.

Perhaps the most readily observed convenient form for bread consumption is the ubiquitous sandwich, which takes slightly different forms in different parts of the world. The sandwich consumption tradition in the UK stretches back many years where many of the 'working-class' lunches were based on sandwiches prepared in the home. Gradually, the convenience of sliced bread, combined with a variety of fillings, moved from the home to mainstream food production. Today the triangular pre-packed sandwich has become an established food source (Figure 1.3), not least in the business community, where longer working hours and shorter lunch breaks often means that sandwiches are eaten at the desk instead of a visit to the company canteen or nearby restaurant. British consumers manage to munch their way through 11.5 billion sandwiches each year and it is said, that if you laid each one end to end they would go around the world about 44 times. In the UK alone in 2017 (www.statista.com/statistics/281823/market-value-of-sandwiches-and-baguettes-in-the-uk-from-2007) around £495 million was spent on the purchase of sandwiches, rolls and baguettes, with sales through retail stores, garages, chemists, high street bakers and coffee shops. In the United States, the sandwich takes a different form, with the type of bread being more similar to rolls in that they contain more sugar. Today, half of all bread products manufactured in the US are sold for the preparation of sandwiches, including those that are associated with well-known fast food outlets. While such sandwiches offer the convenience of 'food on the go', they illustrate the diversity of the nutritional profiles of the products and

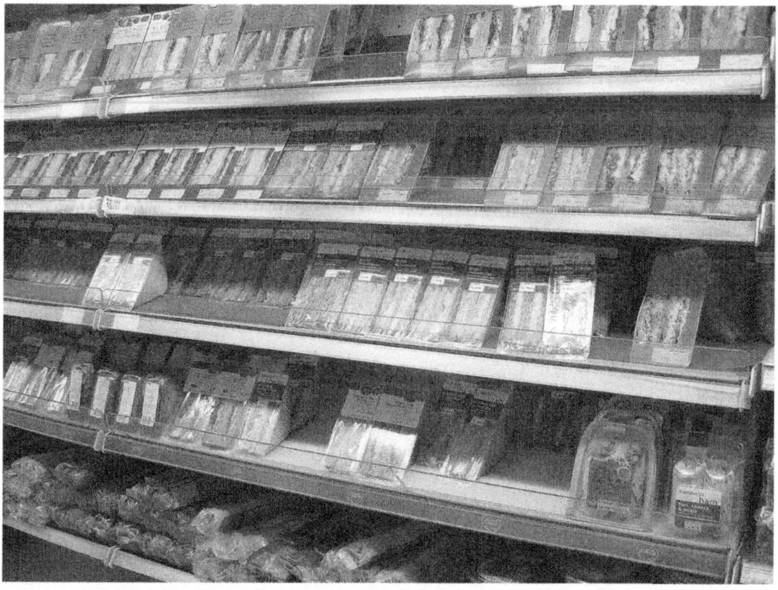

Figure 1.3 Packs of triangular sandwiches.

emphasise the variations in geographical preferences for bakery products (see Chapter 5).

As noted above, sandwiches may be bought in different formats. In the UK and elsewhere, there has been a progressive trend in the bread choice, with the traditional white bread loaf increasingly giving way to variations based on wholemeal, granary, rye, and wheat-germ flour varieties. Bread variants often now include the addition of other non-wheat seeds. In part, this is associated with the desire to confer perceived health benefits for this sector of products. The challenges for the sandwich making industry include, dealing with salt reduction in the bread component (in some parts of the world, especially the UK) and more recently with greater focus on the nutritional value of the fillings. Gone are the days of the restricted choice of only cheese or ham, occasionally garnished with sliced tomato! The increase in the sandwich filling variety has not come without its problems, not least shown by the recent call by Public Health England (PHE) (2018) to reduce the calorie count of sandwiches by 20% by 2024.

1.2 Historical Links Between Baked Products, Nutrition and Health

As knowledge of a contribution of foods to health and well-being of humankind developed, many manufacturers of bakery products have been mindful of their role in delivering improved and relevant nutrition. In some cases, nutritionally enhanced bakery products have been introduced by pioneering individuals, while in others (e.g. fortification) the changes have been government-led. Practical examples related to the value of increasing fibre in the diet can be found in the stories of two bread products developed in the UK in the later nineteenth century. In that period of time the American vegetarian, Sylvester Graham (of Graham cracker fame), insisted on using unsifted wholewheat flour to bake bread, so that consumers could benefit from the laxative properties of the bran. In the UK the same theme was being picked up by Dr Thomas Allinson, who wrote articles on the benefits of vegetarianism and bread, including in 1891 the advantages of eating wholemeal bread (Marchant et al. 2008). At the time he was writing, Dr Allinson considered that no mills produced wholemeal flours to his required standard, so that in 1892 he acquired an interest in a London-based flour mill. He went on to form 'The Natural

Food Company', which traded under the slogan 'health without medicine', a theme which still resounds in many quarters today (though the description of bread as 'natural' would be under greater scrutiny today; see Chapter 8). Allinson wholemeal flour and bread made therefrom, remain available to this day in the UK.

In the preparation of white flour during the nineteenth century, the common practice was to divert bran and wheat-germ components to animal feed. A particular problem is the instability of wheat-germ because of its high fat content which causes it to go rancid relatively quickly. This phenomenon limited its high vitamin and mineral nutritive value for human consumption, a fact quickly recognised by Richard 'Stoney' Smith, a miller in the UK. He found that by heating wheat-germ with steam and a little salt, it would keep much better (Marchant et al. 2008). He established a patent for a bread product based on a wheat-germ treatment method in 1885, later selling the concept to another milling company in 1887. A competition to establish a suitable brand name for the flour and the bread made therefrom, was launched. It was won by a London student, Herbert Grime, who took the Latin for 'strength of man' – *hominis vis* – and shortened it to Hovis. The Hovis Bread Company was formed in 1898 and quickly established itself as a branded bread product, the flour being supplied to bakers along with the method of production and baking pans carrying the Hovis name impressed into the sides of metal pans. The manufacture of the wheat-germ product continues today in the UK, though the Hovis brand name is now applied to a wide range of bread products, including white (Figure 1.4).

Despite the long history of producing fibre rich breads in the UK and elsewhere, the production and consumption of white bread has continued to dominate. As a greater emphasis was progressively placed on the role of dietary fibre throughout the 1980s, bakers began to study potential ways of increasing the fibre content of bread while retaining, as much as possible, the sensory characteristics of white bread. Many fibre rich breads in the 1970s were small in volume, dense in character with a rough mouthfeel and poor keeping qualities. For some sectors of consumers (especially children), these were significant barriers to increasing their fibre consumption using bread products and they were more likely to turn to breakfast cereals. Many of breakfast cereals derive from the interest of nineteenth century physicians, such as John Harvey Kellogg, who was actively engaged in developing and promoting such products so that consumers could

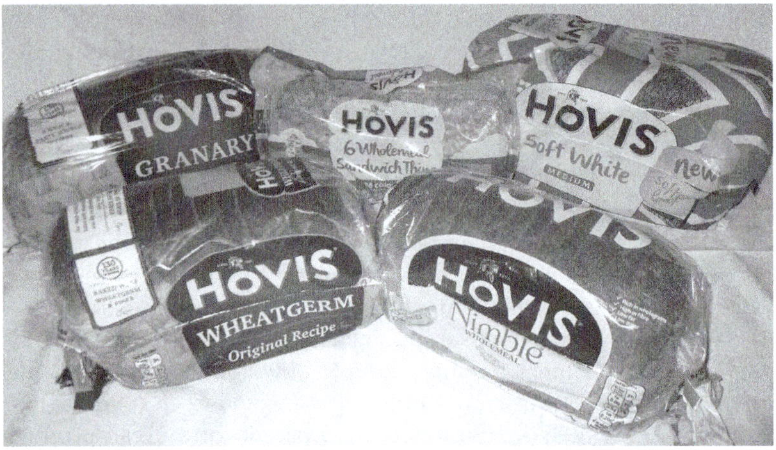

Figure 1.4 Hovis bread products.

benefit from fibre-rich diets. Today the healthy image of breakfast cereals is equally under a degree of nutritional pressure because a number of them are associated with high levels of sugar consumption, an aspect of particular concern for the nutrition of children.

With an increased interest in delivering dietary fibre using bread and other bakery products, technical innovations implemented by millers and bakers were able to deliver new wholemeal and fibre-richer products to consumers and in many parts of the world, there has been a gradual (and important) shift in bread consumption away from white bread. The developments have seen the introduction on non-wheat fibre-rich raw materials, including seeds and other grains, with some extension of the approach to other groups of bakery products. While the move from historical coarse-grained, off-white breads was undoubtedly fuelled in part, by lower prices for flour and bread, there were other factors involved in that progressive switch. Amongst the key factors in delivering increased consumption of non-white breads are improvements to the sensory character of the products. The presence of fibre, certainly as large particles of wheat bran, for many consumers, reduces the sensory pleasure associated with eating bread. In order to deliver more consumer suitable enriched fibre products, developments in flour milling and baking technology were necessary. Such developments combined with appropriate baking technology resulted in the production of fibre-enriched breads using

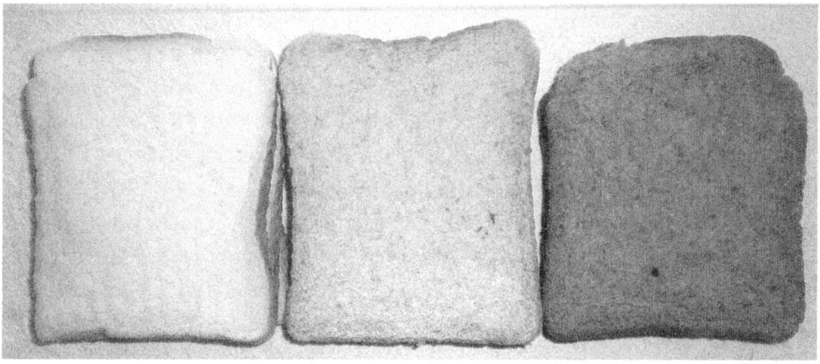

Figure 1.5 Comparison of white and increased fibre breads: left, white bread; middle, 50/50; right, 100% wholemeal.

white and wholemeal flour mixtures For example, in the UK and elsewhere there has been successful growth in products in which the dietary fibre is to some extent less obvious in the bread crumb, such as illustrated in Figure 1.5. In addition to the obvious crumb colour differences, consumers would observe differences in bread volume (lower with wholemeal), crumb texture and eating qualities. Less coloured forms of fibres may also be used to increase the dietary fibre content of breads. Less well-developed, but of increasing interest today, are moves by bakers to limit the contributions of their products to the level of fats and sugars in consumer diets. As will discussed in Chapter 5, consumer geographical sensory preferences will play a significant role in the continuing interest of bakers to making positive contributions to consumer diet and health with their products.

1.3 A Brief History of Concerns Over Fibre, Fat, Sugar and Salt in Baked Products

The science of nutrition is not new; interest in the relationship between foods, diet, and health stretches back many hundreds of years, as recorded in the texts of physicians in antiquity (Gentilcore 2015). As medical knowledge has developed, so has the understanding of the contribution of food nutrients to the human diet and the well-being of consumers. As noted above, physicians of the latter nineteenth century were well-aware of the contribution of fibre in the diet, with a particular interest in the laxative effects and the contribution to regular bowel movements. Medical references often used the term 'roughage' to convey the concept to consumers, along with encouragement to increase the quantity consumed in the diet. It might be said that more recent and increased interest in the contribution of fibre in the diet, intensifies following the studies of Burkitt (1986) and others. While reminding us that prominent physicians of many hundreds of years ago recognised the value of wheat fibre as part of a healthy diet, Burkitt drew attention to the role of fibre in alleviating the 'diseases of western civilisation' such as obesity, diabetes, heart disease, and bowel cancers.

In earlier years, the wheat flour milling industry commonly described and measured fibre under the heading of 'crude' fibre and linked it with cellulose (e.g. Kent-Jones 1939). Crude fibre was to become part of legislative definitions introduced in many parts of the world and even international standards were set, for example the International Association for Cereal Science and Technology (ICC) method 113 (Cauvain 2018). As the study of fibre components and their potential contribution to the diet increased, the needs for more relevant definitions of and analytical methods for measuring fibre became increasingly apparent (McCleary and Prosky 2001), which has led to increasing cooperation between nutritionists and cereals scientists. Today, dietary fibre is better understood and defined, though universal acceptance has still to be achieved. The complexity of defining dietary fibre has not made the task of product development easy for the baking industry. While obviously high levels of fibre are universally associated with wholemeal bread, the position with respect to white or 'brown' breads is less clear. One example of the difficulties which are faced by bakers, revolves around the concept of resistant starch, the definition of which is covered in four different categories. Not all defined forms of resistant starch are present in all forms of bakery products, which hampers the understanding of what might or might not, be analysed as dietary fibre and how this may fit with any related nutritional data and what claims may or may not, be made. In the context of dietary fibre, two recent collaborations between nutritionist and cereal scientists worthy of note are the Healthgrain Forum (https://healthgrain.org) and the Wholegrains Council (https://wholegrainscouncil.org/about-us), both formed to promote greater consumption of dietary fibre through grain-based foods, based on sound science and relevant measurements techniques. Both organisations are active in addressing the negative nutrition and health connotations which have been advocated in recent times and become associated with bread and related products.

Discussions related to the contribution of fat in the diet also have a long and chequered history. Naturally higher in energy density than all of the other major nutrients, the limitation of the level of dietary fat in diets has always been on the nutritionist's agenda. However, in addition to the well-understood energy density contribution, medical research has also focussed on the nature of fats in the diet. Early attention (COMA 1984) focussed on recommendations not only on limiting the proportion of fat in UK diets derived from fat (to 75% of the 1984 intake), but also on a reduction in the consumption of saturated fats. The concepts in the COMA report focussed on improving the ratio of polyunsaturated to saturated fat (P/S ratio). At that time *trans* fatty acids were included with the saturated fats for the purposes of the calculation of the P/S ratio. Typically, at that time, around 4.3% of all fatty acids consumed in the UK diet were in the *trans* form (Burt et al. 1983). Later research (e.g. Mozaffarian et al. 2006) was to highlight the role of *trans* fatty acids with respect to the incidence of cardiovascular disease and add to growing concerns over the negative roles of the various types of fat in consumers' diets. Concerns linking the contribution of dietary saturated fat to high levels of cholesterol in the bloodstream, have also received much attention in the nutrition and medical fields, though it is necessary to distinguish between the so-called 'good' and 'bad' forms of cholesterol; known respectively as high density lipoprotein (HDL) and low density lipoprotein (LDL) because of the combination of lipid (fat) and proteins which form in the bloodstream.

Possibly the seminal work which altered nutritionists' views of the medical dangers of excessive consumption of sugar in the diet, was that produced by John Yudkin, a Professor in the Department of Nutrition at Queen Elizabeth College, London. First published in 1972 and later republished a number of times (Yudkin 2016), *Pure, White and Deadly: How Sugar is Killing Us and What We Can Do to Stop it,* set the scene for much of the research on sugars in the diet in the last 40 years or so (see for example, Goran et al. 2015). Ground-breaking as Yudkin's treatise was, it did little to stop the increasing consumption of sugar in the years which followed its initial publication. Sugars provide a readily assimilated source of energy and induce sensory pleasure during consumption. However, Mintz (1985) identified that the desire of sweetness in the human diet is not innate, and also drew attention to historical and social factors which may have contributed to the significantly and progressively increasing consumption of sugar and sugar-containing foods. Lustig et al. (2012) argued that the negative health aspects of excess consumption of sugars were so serious that added sweeteners should be controlled in a similar manner to that of alcohol. The role of food companies in 'promoting' sugar consumption was recently discussed by McLennan et al. (2015) who drew attention to role of advertising and brand image in sugar-containing foods. In doing so, they have highlighted the key and responsible role that food producers can play in delivering improved nutrition and health.

While in most recent years there has been a strong focus on levels of salt in consumers' diets and the contribution that bakery products might make in this context, medical concerns regarding salt and health are not entirely new. Perhaps the most active geographic area has been the UK, with the UK's Food Standards Agency and Department of Health taking a particular interest in lowering the level of salt in bread following a survey of sodium in the diet in the late 1980s (Gregory et al. 1990). Such surveys coincided with increased medical concerns being raised regarding the contribution of sodium to high blood pressure and other potential negative effects on health, as outlined by a number of medical practitioners, including extensive studies by He and MacGregor (2007). The formation in the UK of a Committee for Action on Salt and Health (CASH) led to a series of consultations between representatives of the UK baking industry through the Federation of Bakers and the UK Food Standards Agency which established a series of targets for salt reduction in bread and other fermented products, according to an agreed timetable. This collaboration was voluntary in nature and with the support of the UK baking industry, was to lead to significant reductions in the contribution of bread and fermented products for dietary sodium levels. Using the collaborative principles established with bread, the UK baking industry was to extend its actions to reducing dietary sodium levels in other baked products. In some parts of the world the process of salt reduction has been voluntary, though in others it has been mandatory in nature, not least by taking into account the UK's lead on this topic.

1.4 Current Nutrition and Health Concerns

In many ways the current concerns regarding the nutrition and health contributions of bakery products have become subsumed in the greater concern regarding the dramatic increase in the proportion of individuals in modern populations who may be classified as overweight or obese. It is sometimes difficult for the average person to separate problems of overweight from associated medical conditions because there is no certain causal relationship. Individuals who are overweight may well live apparent healthy lives, while individuals with medical conditions, such as type II diabetes, are not always overweight. Nevertheless, there is significant global concern and medical evidence to encourage changes in the dietary habits of many individuals to reduce body mass and in doing so, to make positive contributions to their health and well-being. While the position regarding adults is of great concern, that for children is alarming (see for example data presented in Delpeuch et al. 2009). Overweight and obesity are increasingly linked with health problems such as type II diabetes, coronary heart disease, high blood pressure, strokes, some cancers, liver disease, gallstones, osteoarthritis, respiratory problems, sleep apnoea, infertility, and mental illnesses, such as clinical depression. However, the increase in the incidence of the medical conditions described above cannot be solely ascribed to obesity. Lustig et al. (2012) noted that 40% of normal weight individuals can develop these medical conditions, while 20% of obese individuals have normal metabolism. Nevertheless it is globally recognised that the overall increase in average individual body mass is most often associated with the increased prevalence of the common medical conditions noted above and increasingly in turn, this places greater pressures on health services and contributes to the ever-increasing medical costs.

Many causes are cited for the increasing body mass of many individuals. They are somewhat emotively stated to include, often without clear definition or supporting evidence:

- Diseases of civilised societies and westernised diets.
- Changes in the pattern of food consumption way from ‘traditional’ diets (for example, see data in Delpeuch et al. 2009).
- A rise in the consumption of so-called convenience and ‘highly processed’ foods.

Collectively such statements have identified that many individuals have a high energy intake (put simply, they eat too much) and that often the foods that they consume are high in fat, sugar and salt. In addition many modern diets are considered to be low in fibre and in the consumption of fruit and vegetables. A contributing factor to global obesity is related to changes in lifestyles, which commonly includes less physical exercise than was the case in the past. Cordain et al. (2005) provide a comprehensive review of the evolution of the 'so-called' Western diet and current health indications. It perhaps too simplistic to use the terms civilised or Westernised diets, since the diet most commonly associated with the Mediterranean world (http://mediterradiet.org/nutrition/mediterranean_diet_pyramid) is often seen in a virtuous light and associated with the potential for weight loss. However, the evidence for some of the 'healthy' claims associated with the Mediterranean diet are equivocal and many elements of the diet are not relevant to the development of nutritionally enhanced bakery products.

In the global context of current health and lifestyle concerns, the role of the food manufacturer has inevitably been highlighted and examined in some detail. While the consumers' choice of foods have a strong regional and traditional bias, globalisation of some products has introduced common themes across the world. To some extent this is true for bakery products which are commonly manufactured and consumed in geographical locations which have no history of wheat-based agriculture. The manufacture of bakery products in large parts of the world is based on the importation of wheat with the end-products competing in the local marketplace against more traditional foods. There are geographical variations in the composition of similarly named bakery products, such as bread, which have developed based on the historical introduction of baking technology and consumer preferences (for a more detailed discussion see Chapter 5). However, in the context of current global health concerns, a number of common features can be identified related to high levels of salt, fat, sugar and, in many cases, low levels of dietary fibre. Reformulating bakery products to contribute to reducing the problems of global obesity is not a simple task, but the need of baking industries around the world to make positive contributions has been recognised and accepted.

Nutrition and food-health related studies are important for improving the well-being of humankind (Carlisle and Hanlon 2014). However, the results of many nutritional studies may be equivocal; these raise uncertainties in the minds of food manufacturers as to the validity and relevance of the information which they receive. As will be discussed in Chapter 8, the understanding and application of nutrition and health-studies may not be helped by the manner in which they are sometimes communicated through the media and marketing (Jackson et al. 2014), or as presented by special interest groups (Cauvain 2003). Such discussions further compound uncertainties in the food industry as to which nutritional objectives should be addressed, how they should be delivered, and how they should be communicated. Not all of the views expressed regarding the nutritional value of bread and other bakery products have a sound scientific basis, with apocryphal information repeated without critical question. The persistent myth that bread is fattening is one example, not least because of its 'high' carbohydrate content. As early as the 1950s medical advice for weight loss focussed on reduced carbohydrate intake, with potatoes and bread being given as examples. For some years now, nutritionists have been working to show the benefits of consuming wholemeal bread, a low-fat food that is full of nourishment, with complex sugars that are assimilated slowly by the body. Enriched with bran and wheat-germ delivering vitamins and minerals, it comes packed with dietary fibre that benefits the intestinal tract.

1.5 Improving the Micronutrient Content of Wheat-Based Products

While there is a long history of materials being added to flour, the early focus was more on improving the baking quality of the flour rather than its nutritional qualities. Indeed some of the so-called 'improvements' had potentially negative health connotations because of a lack of relevant knowledge. On occasions, additions were more likely to be associated with profit-driven motives and fell in the definition of adulteration rather than improvement. Fortunately the flour milling and baking industries have long put such dubious practices behind them; in more recent times many additions to flour and baked products are directly related to improving nutritional profiles. An early example of the practice of flour fortification to improve nutrition and health of whole populations, is that implemented in the UK during the 1940s. With the advent of conflict in Europe and the dependence of the UK on supplies of imported wheat for bread production, the UK Accessory Food Factors Committee of the Medical Research Council made important recommendations to conserve supplies and improve the nutritional value of bread and flour. The extraction rate in the mill was raised to 85%, with restrictions in the use of bleaching agents which resulted in bread with a dull and firm crumb. More importantly they proposed that a calcium salt should be added to flour during its manufacture, since those food rich in calcium, such as milk and cheese were expected to be in short supply. Calcium carbonate was chosen, and acetic acid was added to prevent 'rope' formation, rope being a bacterial infection of bread, encouraged by the calcium carbonate addition. Some time after, iron and vitamin fortification were added and despite periodic reviews (at the time of writing), such additions remain mandatory in white flours produced in the UK. Wholemeal flours are not subject to the mandatory need for fortification.

Fortification may be defined as adding vitamins and minerals to foods to prevent nutritional deficiencies and since the consumption in various forms of grains such as wheat, maize, and rice is widespread, these are often the chosen vehicles for delivering improved nutrition with the aim of disease prevention, strengthening of the immune system, and improved productivity and cognitive development. Fortification is considered to be successful because it makes frequently eaten foods more nutritious without relying on consumers to change their dietary habits or food choices. The United Nations (2017) continues to consider that the fortification of commonly eaten grains as an important step towards addressing these. Twelve vitamins and minerals are suggested for use for flour and rice fortification globally, with each country setting its own standards and choosing specific nutrients to meet its population needs.

Common materials used for fortification and their potential contributions to human health and well-being include:

- Iron, which helps prevent nutritional anaemia.
- Folic acid (vitamin B9), reduces the risk of severe birth defects of the brain and spine.
- Zinc, helps childhood development, strengthens immune systems and lessens complications from diarrhoea.
- Niacin (vitamin B3), prevents the skin disease pellagra.
- Riboflavin (vitamin B2), helps with metabolism of fats, carbohydrates and proteins.

- Thiamine (vitamin B1), prevents the nervous system disease beriberi.
- Vitamin B12, helps maintain brain and nervous system functions.
- Vitamin D, helps the absorption calcium and improves bone health.
- Vitamin A, deficiencies contribute to childhood blindness and reduce the ability of an individual to fight infections.
- Calcium, contributes to bone strength, helps transmit nerve messages and assists with muscle function and blood clotting.
- Selenium, helps with reproduction and thyroid gland functions.
- Vitamin B6, needed to support the enzyme reactions involved in food metabolism.

For more detailed information on the principles and practices associated with food fortification, readers are referred elsewhere; for example, the Food Fortification Initiative at www.ffinetwork.org/

The fortification of raw materials for the manufacture of baked products has included the introduction of folic acid in a number of geographical areas. Folic acid fortification reduces the risk for women giving birth to babies with neural tube defects. This particular fortification has not been universally accepted, with countries such as Australia and New Zealand introducing mandatory fortification with folic acid, while the subject remains (at the time of writing) under discussion in the UK. While the medical evidence may be clear about the risks for neural tube defects, concerns in some parts of the world (e.g. the UK) remain regarding potential negative health benefits related to the masking of certain vitamin deficiencies in some sectors of communities. The introduction of iodised salt is another example of differing views on the mandatory fortification of a food raw material.

1.6 Conclusions

Bakery products are a diverse group of food products with a history of production which in the case of bread, stretches back to the early days of agricultural developments in prehistory. While the origins of grain-based bakery products are closely associated with those geographic areas where wheat and other grains can be grown, bakery products are manufactured and consumed in all countries of the world. The addition of ingredients like salt, fat and sugar, not only contributed to taste and texture, but were integral in developing products like cakes, cookies (biscuits) and pastries. The early development of such products was undoubtedly associated with the delivery of sensory pleasure. While bread remained a staple food source for many parts of the population, cakes, cookies and pastries were mostly associated with the higher echelons of societies. As the manufacture of bakery products became more industrialised and the cost of raw materials like sugar fell, the consumption of cakes, cookies and pastries increased, though they were not eaten as regularly as bread.

The current concerns regarding health and diet are commonly associated with the significant rise in the average body mass of individuals. The phenomenon is global and often associated with the availability and consumption of modern processed foods, which includes bakery products. Concerns over the healthiness of bakery products stretch back to the nineteenth century and include the development of new bakery products with increased health benefits. Today, in many communities, the consumption bread and other bakery products is less about the need to achieve an adequate energy intake and more about the sensory pleasures involved in eating such products.

Because of their widespread consumption, it is inevitable that bakery products have attracted the attention of nutritionists and dieticians. In bread, an initial focus was on the contribution that the recipe salt makes to dietary sodium intake, with significant activity in some geographical areas leading to a reduction in the levels used in production. The recognition that bread can make significant contributions to dietary fibre is far from new, but the switch to the consumption of non-white breads has really only increased in the last 10–15 years. Not that the change in the consumption pattern is universal, with white bread continuing to be the product of choice in many parts of the world. Less well advanced, are moves to limit sugar and fat in non-bread bakery products, such as cookies, cakes and pastries. The difficulties in reformulating such products are in some ways more challenging than those with bread.

The fortification of wheat flour with micronutrients has an established history and has been, and continues to be, used in a significant number of countries. The widespread production and ubiquitous consumption of wheat-based products makes products like bread, the ideal vehicles for improving the nutrition of major sectors of populations.

References

Arranz-Otaegui, A., Gonzalez Carretero, L., Ramsey, M.N. et al. (2018). Archaeobotanical evidence reveals the origins of bread 14,400 years ago in northeastern Jordan. *Proceedings of the National Academy of Sciences of the United States of America* https://doi.org/10.1073/pnas.1801071115.

Ashton, J. (1904). *The History of Bread from Pre-Historic to Modern Times*. London, UK: Religious Tract Society.

Bailey, A. (1975). *The Blessings of Bread*. London, UK: Paddington Press.

Burkitt, D.P. (1986). Forward. In: *Dietary Fiber: Basic and Clinical Aspects* (ed. G.V. Vahouny and D. Kritchevsky), ix–xii. New York: Plenum Press.

Burt, R., Buss, D.H., and Kirk, R.S. (1983). Fatty acids and sterols in the British diet. *Proceedings of the Nutrition Society* 42: 71A.

Carlisle, S. and Hanlon, P. (2014). Connecting food, well-being and environmental sustainability. *Critical Public Health* 24 (4): 405–417.

Cauvain, S.P. (2003). Bread industry and consumer expectations regarding organic bakery products in the European Union [in German]. *Getreide, Mehl & Brot* 57: 100–107.

Cauvain, S.P. (2015). *Technology of Breadmaking*, 3e. Cham Heidelberg, Switzerland: Springer International Publishing.

Cauvain, S.P. (2018). *The ICC Handbook of Cereals, Flour, Dough & Product Testing: Methods and Applications*. Lancaster, PA: DESTech Publications.

Committee on Medical Aspect of Food Policy – COMA (1984) *Diet and Cardiovascular Disease*. Report of the Panel on Diet in Relation to Cardiovascular Disease. Department of Health and Social Security. Report on Health Subjects 28. London: HMSO.

Cordain, L., Eaton, S.B., Sebastian, A. et al. (2005). Origins and evolution of the Western diet: health implication for the 21st century. *American Journal of Clinical Nutrition* 81: 341–354.

Delpeuch, F., Maire, B., Monnier, E., and Holdswort, M. (2009). *Globesity: A Planet out of Control?* London: Earthscan.

Gentilcore, D. (2015). *Food and Health in Early Modern Europe*. London: Bloomsbury Academic.

Goran, M.I., Tappy, L., and Le, K.-A. (2015). *Dietary Sugars and Health*. Boca Raton, FL: Taylor and Francis Group.

Gregory, J., Foster, K., Tyler, H., and Wiseman, M. (1990). *The Dietary and Nutrition Survey of British Adults*. London: HMSO.

He, J.J. and MacGregor, G.A. (2007). Dietary salt, high blood pressure and other harmful effects on health. In: *Reducing Salt in Foods: Practical Strategies* (ed. D. Kilcast and F. Angus), 18–54. Cambridge, UK: Woodhead Publishing.

Jackson, M., Harrison, P., Swinburn, B., and Lawrence, M. (2014). Unhealthy food, integrated marketing communication and power: a critical analysis. *Critical Public Health* 24 (4): 489–505.

Kent-Jones, D.W. (1939). *Modern Cereal Chemistry*, 3e. Liverpool, UK: The Northern Publishing Co.

Lustig, R.H., Schmidt, L.A., and Brindis, C.D. (2012). The toxic truth about sugar. *Nature* 482: 27–29.

Marchant, J., Reuben, B., and Alcock, J. (2008). *Bread: A Slice History*. Stroud, UK: The History Press.

McCleary, B. and Prosky, L. (2001). *Advanced Dietary Fibre Technology*. Oxford, UK: Blackwell Science.

McLennan, A.K., Ulijaszek, S.J., and Eli, K. (2015). Social aspects of dietary sugars. In: *Dietary Sugars and Health* (ed. M.I. Goran, L. Tappy and K.-A. Le), 1–11. Boca Raton, FL: Taylor and Francis Group.

Mintz, S.W. (1985). *Sweetness and Power: The Place of Sugar in Modern History*. New York, NY: Penguin Books.

Mozaffarian, D., Katan, M.B., Ascherio, A. et al. (2006). *Trans* fatty acids and cardiovascular disease. *New England Journal of Medicine* 354: 1601–1613.

Public Health England (2018). *Calorie Reduction: The Scope and Ambition for Action*. London: PHE Publications www.gov.uk/government/publications/calorie-reduction-the-scope-and-ambition-for-action.

Samuel, D. (1999). Bread making and social interactions at the Amarna Workmen's village, Egypt. *World Archaeology* 31 (1): 121–144.

Toussaint-Samat, M. (1992). *A History of Food*. Oxford, UK: Blackwell Publishing.

Ucko, P.J. and Dimbleby, G.W. (1969). *The Domestication and Exploitation of Plants and Animals*. London: UK: Gerald Duckworth.

United Nations (2017) https://unstats.un.org/sdgs/files/report/2017/TheSustainableDevelopmentGoalsReport2017.pdf/

Yudkin, J. (2016). *Pure, White and Deadly: How Sugar Is Killing Us and What We Can Do to Stop It*. London: Penguin Ransom House.

2

Summary of the Manufacture of Bakery Products and Their Key Characteristics

2.1 Introduction

There are no clear definitions as to what constitutes a bakery product, or the processes by which they are made. Even the basic assumption that bakery products will be based on the use of wheat flour in their manufacture is questionable. The wide variety of what constitutes a bakery product is the result of the evolutionary processes by which we have arrived at the current family of bakery products. Within the family of products generally regarded as belonging to a bakery, it has become common to describe various sub-classes, largely using composite definitions based on ingredients, recipes, and final product characteristics. In some cases, a process element may be included in the sub-class description, but this is not common.

Commonly the main sub-classes of bakery products are defined as:

- Bread and fermented goods.
- Biscuits, cookies, and crackers.
- Cakes and sponges.
- Pastries.

In the context of this work, the diagram used by Cauvain and Young (2006a) and reproduced here with some modification (Figure 2.1), provides a useful means of identifying sub-classes of bakery products. In their approach Cauvain and Young plotted bakery sub-classes using ratios of recipe sugar to flour and fat to flour. They did so in the context of highlighting the impact of these ingredients on the formation of a gluten network, or its limitation

Baking Technology and Nutrition: Towards a Healthier World, First Edition.
Stanley P. Cauvain and Rosie H. Clark.

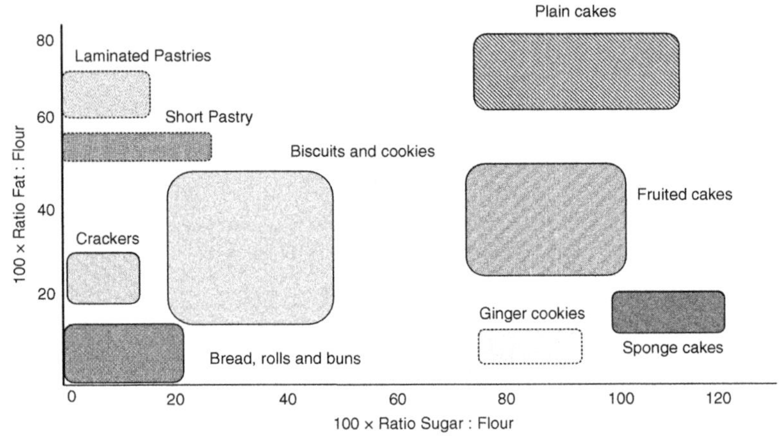

Figure 2.1 Sub-classes of bakery products.

from the addition of fats and sugars; key roles for these ingredients have significant implications for the manufacture of nutritionally enhanced bakery products. The same authors also referred to the role and adaptation of processing technology to deliver specific baked product characteristics. Such discussions highlight one of the main premises of this work, namely, that reductions in functional ingredients, such as fat and sugar in bakery products, are only likely to be achieved through an understanding of the complex ingredient–recipe–process interactions involved. Cauvain and Young (2008) also highlighted the critical role that water plays, not only in forming the sub-classes of bakery products, but also the key contribution that moisture makes to the shelf-life and textural characteristics of baked products.

In Figure 2.2 various sub-classes of bakery products are plotted based on the relationship between final product moisture and water activity. While it is true that moisture content and product water activity are linked (higher moisture levels yield higher water activity and vice versa), there are many recipe factors which can influence water activity without significant changes in product moisture content as discussed by Cauvain and Young (2008). There may also be a process element associated with moisture losses during baking, with more oven heat input resulting in higher water losses and therefore lower product moistures. Equally important for baked products is the contribution of moisture to the formation of particular product

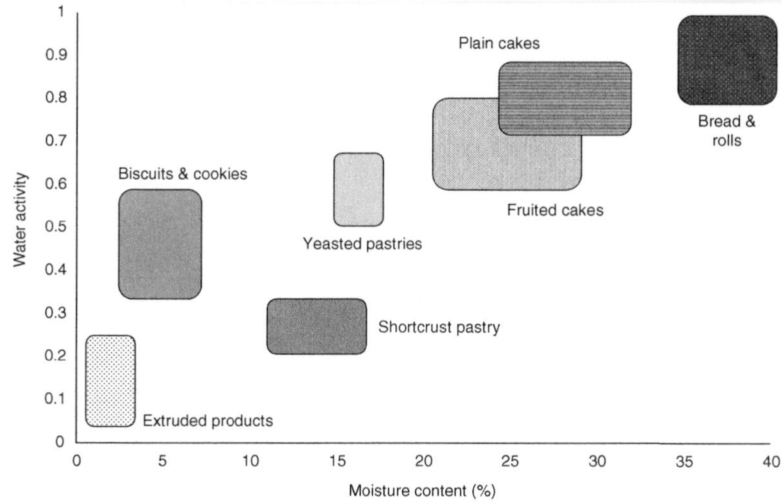

Figure 2.2 Relationship between final product moisture and water activity for various bakery products.

textures during processing and in the final product. A summary of the descriptors often used with baked products texture and their overall relationship with product moisture is illustrated in Figure 2.3. Broadly speaking, product textures become softer as moisture content rises but the manner in which the texture is formed also has an influence, with aerated structures also contributing to soft eating characters. Some products, e.g. bread, are based on a mixture of textures, with the low moisture content on the crust making it 'crisp' eating, while the high moisture of the crumb contributes to its soft eating character. An often ignored contribution of water in determining the final product texture, is its role in forming aerated structures; for example, in contributing to gluten formation during dough mixing.

2.2 A Synopsis of Common Bread and Fermented Product Types, and Their Manufacturing Processes

Key characteristics of the bread and fermented product sub-class are that the recipes contain yeast (for dough inflation – gas production) and that a strong gluten network is formed in the dough by which to

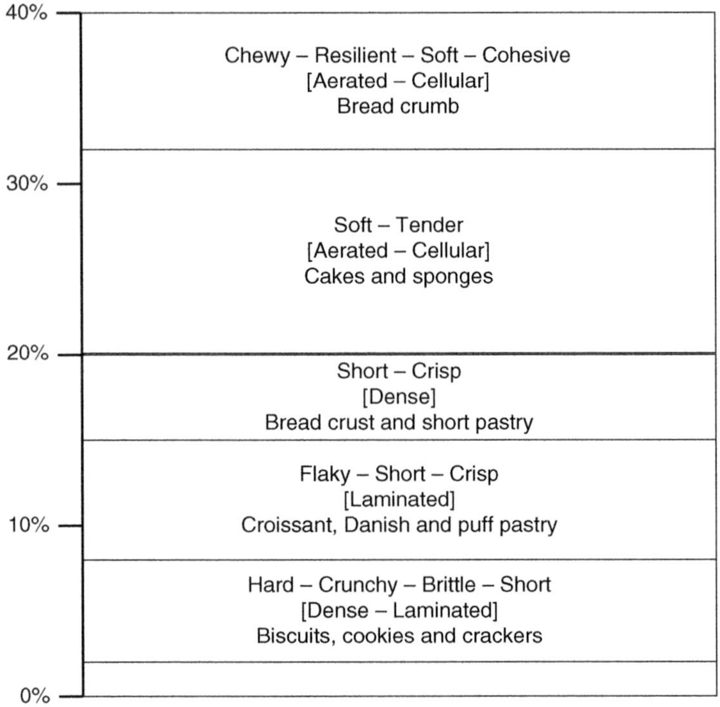

Figure 2.3 Relationship between final product moisture and eating quality.

trap carbon dioxide gas from yeast fermentation. This gluten network is deliberately formed through the input of energy during mixing (Cauvain 2015) and confers on the dough a property commonly referred to as 'gas retention'. The transition from dough to bread is referred to as a 'foam to sponge' conversion, with the foam comprising gas bubbles trapped in the gluten matrix formed during mixing (Dobraszczyk et al. 2001; Campbell and Martin 2012; Wilde 2012). The input of heat and loss of moisture during baking in the oven creates the sponge. It is important to recognise that the concept of a foam to sponge conversion is not a single discrete event in the manufacture of bread and fermented products, but happens gradually as the heat front in the oven travels from the dough piece surface to its centre. Thus, it is important to recognise the role that heat transfer makes in delivering the final structure and the impact of ingredients (such as sugar) on the temperature, and by definition the time, at which the transition is made in the oven.

A wide range of bread products are manufactured around the world which may be broadly classified as:

- Pan breads, with the dough pieces being placed in pans for proving and baking.
- Hearth or oven-bottom breads, with the dough piece being baked on the hearth of the oven, or on flat or shaped trays.
- Rolls and buns, in which the addition of fat and sugar modifies the final product eating character and sensory shelf-life.

The creation of a sponge structure in the final product delivers the most commonly sought character in all breads and fermented products, namely a soft and resilient crumb with some chewiness. These crumb characteristics are common, even if the crust character varies from thin and soft (e.g. sandwich bread) to hard and crusty (e.g. baguette). Even fermented products which are not baked in an oven and lack a coloured crust, e.g. steamed bread and buns (Huang 2014), are expected to have a soft, resilient, and chewy crumb.

2.3 The Bread Manufacturing Processes

There are a wide variety of breadmaking processes in use around the world. Essentially, they all involve the mixing of wheat flour, yeast, salt, and other functional ingredients with water. The latter hydrates the proteins and damaged starch, and with the input (at different levels) of mechanical work (even hand mixing delivers energy to the dough during mixing) a visco-elastic gluten network is developed which allows the entrapment of carbon dioxide gas from yeast fermentation. After the bulk dough is mixed, the preparation and shaping of individual dough pieces follows, with continued fermentation in the prover and finally a heat-setting step in the oven (Cauvain 2001). The different classes of breadmaking processes vary most in the manner in which the dough ingredients are mixed and the gluten network is developed. The main breadmaking processes were divided into five broad groups by Cauvain (2015):

- Sour-dough processes.
- Straight dough bulk fermentation.
- Sponge and dough.
- Rapid processing (no-time dough).
- Mechanical dough development.

2.3.1 Sour-Dough Processes

More recently, the term 'artisan' has been coined to label the methods used to manufacture sour dough processes. In some cases, very specific descriptors, e.g. San Francisco sour dough, may be used to identify the method (not the location) by which the bread has been produced (Gobbetti and Ganzle 2013). Considered by some to be the most traditional of breadmaking processes, sour dough processes commonly only use flour, water, salt and yeast and in some variations, even the latter may be omitted and the presence of wild yeast and lactic acid bacteria naturally present in the flour and from the atmosphere, are used as the means of generating the required carbon dioxide gas during fermentation. In this sub-group of processes, the development of a 'mother' dough is essential, with small portions of it being taking for subsequent bread production. Fermentation periods associated with sponges and the final bulk doughs, stretch for many hours according to the flavour profile required in the final products. Mixing may be carried out by hand or with a machine, with dough processing and baking following much the standard pattern as with other types of breadmaking process. What sets this type of bread process apart from others, is the deliberate development of strongly acidic flavours in the final products, commonly attributable to lactic and acetic acids (Calvel et al. 2001; Schunemann and Treu 2001; Cauvain 2016a). Both wheat and rye flours may be used, with a strong traditional bias towards the latter in northern Europe and Scandinavia. The acidic flavour may be adjusted by changing dough fermentation conditions to favour either lactic or acetic sour notes in the baked bread.

2.3.2 Straight Dough Bulk Fermentation

Another breadmaking method with a long history, the essential features of bulk fermentation (sometimes called long fermentation) can be summed up as follows:

- mixing of the ingredients to form an homogeneous dough;
- resting of the dough so formed in bulk for a prescribed time (floor-time), commonly many hours. The length of fermentation time used for optimum bread quality depends on flour quality, yeast level, dough temperature and the bread variety being produced;

- part-way through the prescribed bulk fermentation period there may be a remixing of the dough (a 'knock-back');
- after fermentation the bulk dough is divided and processed as unit pieces in the common manner described above.

Dough mixing is usually carried out with low-speed mixing machines and dough development is almost completely limited to that achieved by the natural enzymic processes which take place during the bulk fermentation period. The further input of energy during the 'knock-back' (effectively a limited re-mix of the dough) makes a contribution to final dough development. The control of factors which affect the bulk fermentation process (i.e. time, temperature, and yeast level) play a significant role in determining product quality because they collectively affect the rate and extent of gluten network modification during the prescribed fermentation period. The length of the bulk fermentation period may vary from 1 to 16 hours depending on the requirements of the baker; commonly periods of 2–4 hours are used especially in larger, industrial-scale bakeries.

2.3.3 Sponge and Dough

Elements of sponge and dough processes are similar to those for bulk fermentation, in that a prolonged period of fermentation is required to effect physical and chemical changes in the dough. In a sponge and dough process, this is achieved by the thorough fermentation of part of the dough ingredients rather than all of them, as is the case with bulk fermentation. The key features of sponge and dough processes may be summarised as:

- the mixing of part of the total quantity of flour (typically 15–40% of the recipe flour weight), water, and other ingredients from the formulation to form the sponge;
- bulk fermentation of the sponge for a prescribed time (floor-time), typically 2–24 hours and commonly under defined temperature conditions;
- mixing of the sponge with the remainder of the ingredients to form an homogenous dough;
- immediate processing of the final dough (though in some variations a limited period of further bulk fermentation may be used).

In the UK, sponge and dough formation tends to be a low-speed process carried out with low-speed mixing machines, while in North

America more intense mixing is given to the sponge and the subsequent dough using horizontal bar mixers. The main roles of the sponge are to modify the flavour of the final product (more acidic) and to contribute to the development of the final dough through the modification of its rheological properties, usually from natural enzymic processes, though gluten-modifying ingredients may also be used.

2.3.4 Rapid Processing (No-Time Dough)

This heading covers a multitude of slightly different breadmaking systems, each of which has evolved based on different combinations of raw materials, active ingredients, mixing equipment and processing methods. A common element within this process group is the inclusion of improvers to assist in dough development and the reduction of any individual fermentation period, in bulk or as divided pieces (but not including proof) to significantly less than one hour. In many process variations, the bulk dough will move directly from the mixing bowl to the divider without a resting period (no-time). Spiral and similar mixing machines are most commonly used in a single dough preparation stage and the mechanical energy imparted to the dough during mixing is an important element of dough development.

2.3.5 Mechanical Dough Development

The common elements of this group of breadmaking processes are that there is no deliberate fermentation period in bulk and that dough development is achieved almost entirely in the mixing machine, often in combination with a suitable dough oxidising agent. After leaving the mixer the bulk dough is divided and processed without delay, and the transition from flour to bread may be achieved in around two hours.

Perhaps the best known and most widely used of the mechanical dough development processes is the one launched in the UK in 1961 – the Chorleywood Bread Process (CBP) which is in use in many counties around the world today (Cauvain and Young 2006b). The essential features of the CBP remain largely unchanged since its introduction and they are:

- mixing and dough development in a single operation, lasting between two and five minutes to a fixed energy input per kg of dough in the mixer;

- the addition of an oxidising improver above that added in the flour mill, now most commonly ascorbic acid;
- the addition of extra water to adjust dough consistency for processing to be comparable with that from bulk fermentation;
- the addition of extra yeast to maintain final proof times to be comparable with those obtained with bulk fermented doughs;
- the inclusion of a high melting point fat, emulsifier, or fat and emulsifier combination;
- the control of mixer headspace atmosphere to achieve given bread cell structures.

The role that energy plays in optimising bread quality during mechanical dough development is particularly important and a common practice with CBP is to mix to a fixed energy level per kilogram of dough in the mixer. When first introduced, optimum energy levels quickly became standardised at 11 W-h kg^{-1} dough (5 W-h lb), but with changing wheat varieties over the 50 years or so since its introduction, it has now become more common to vary the energy input according to flour qualities. In general, high protein flours yield a stronger gluten network and so require higher energy input in order to optimise dough development, with higher energy input comes greater temperature rise during the mixing cycle (Cauvain and Young 2006b).

One important aspect of the CBP that is not readily available in other breadmaking processes, is the potential for the direct control of the cell structure in the final bread through the adjustment of the headspace pressure during the mixing cycle. Pressures below atmospheric tend to give fine cell structure (i.e. smaller cell sizes) while those above atmospheric pressures give more open cell structures (i.e. larger cell sizes). The versatility of the CBP has been increased with the introduction of mixers with the capability of moving from one pressure to another sequentially during the mixing cycle (Cauvain 2015). This versatility enables a variety of bread types to be made from the same dough formulation and processing equipment (Cauvain 1994).

2.3.6 Dough Processing from Divider to Prover

Whatever the process used to prepare a dough for breadmaking, a point is reached when the bulk of the dough needs to be divided into a number of different unit sizes for further processing. The processing of the unit-sized dough pieces is usually carried out as a series of shaping operations, often with short rest periods (first or intermediate proof) between individual operations to adjust the rheological properties of the dough in order to yield the desired bread qualities. A wide range of processing equipment is available for the tasks associated with dough processing (Cauvain 2015) but in all cases during these moulding and processing stages, the rheological properties of the dough are critical and bakers will seek to optimise these by appropriate choice of recipe ingredients, dough development, and adjustment of added dough water levels (Cauvain et al. 2015).

2.3.7 Expansion in the Prover and Structure Setting in the Oven

The expansion and setting of dough pieces to two or three times their original size marks the transformation from dough to bread. At the heart of this transition are two fundamental processes which underpin the production of all fermented products; gas production and gas retention (Cauvain 2015). As noted above, the production of carbon dioxide by the bakers' yeast in the dough is responsible for the gas production component, while the developed gluten network is responsible for the gas retention component of the dough. In the prover, heat and humidity are introduced to further stimulate gas production by the yeast and the small gas bubbles that are trapped in the gluten network begin to expand, so that the dough pieces usually increase to at least twice their original size (Cauvain 2015). Further expansion of the gas bubbles takes place in the early stages of baking and at this time the ability of the dough to retain the carbon dioxide gas being produced before the yeast is inactivated, the release of dissolved carbon dioxide, the steam being generated and the thermal expansion of all the trapped gases, are dependent on the gas retention properties of the dough. Usually doughs with good gas retention show 'oven spring,' that is the size of the baked loaf is greater than the size of the proved dough piece when it entered the oven.

2.4 A Synopsis of Biscuit, Cookie and Cracker Types and Their Manufacturing Processes

Biscuits and cookies may be separated into five broad categories; hard-dough semi-sweet, rotary-moulded short-dough, wire-cut cookie, crackers, and wafers (Cauvain 2016b). The individual groups of biscuits and cookies may be distinguished from one another according to the degree to which gluten development occurs, or is desirable, as well as on the basis of the type of equipment used in their production. The key elements of the groups are summarised in Table 2.1. In all cases the levels of water used in the mixing of the biscuit dough are low by comparison with bread dough, partly to limit the formation of gluten during mixing and partly to reduce the amount of water that needs to be driven-off during baking to ensure that the products have the hard-eating qualities which are a key characteristic of products in this group. Typically, the baked moisture contents of biscuits, cookies, and crackers fall well below 10% and this contributes to their hard and crisp eating characteristics, and long shelf-life. With their low moisture content and water activities, such products do not commonly have problems with mould growth, provided that they are not allowed to absorb water from the atmosphere or from other sources.

The viscosity (consistency) of biscuit and cookie doughs plays a very important part in the choice and operation of a particular production process. In the case of short- and cookie-doughs, gluten development needs to be limited so that the shaping and forming processes for individual pieces can be easily accomplished, and to avoid changes in biscuit shape (e.g. shrinkage) after forming and

Table 2.1 Key elements of biscuit and cookie types.

Product	Manufacturing form	Gluten formation (by comparison with bread dough)	Texture and eating qualities
Crackers and other laminated biscuits	Sheeted, laminated, and cut dough	Modest	Brittle and flaky
Semi-sweet	Sheeted and cut dough	Limited	Hard
Short dough	Rotary moulded dough	None	Short and sweet
Cookies	Rotary moulded, rout press, wire-cut deposited dough	None	Short and tender
Wafers	Deposited batter	None	Short and brittle

during baking. In addition to the effects of recipe ingredients and their levels, the dough mixing method may be modified in an attempt to limit gluten formation. The most common variation is called 'creaming' because all the ingredients, except the flour and a few other non-functional ingredients, are first mixed together. The sugars and other materials are dissolved in the recipe water and the resulting solution becomes dispersed in the fat. At this stage the mixture has a creamy-white colour and a soft consistency, hence the popular name for this type of mixing process. Finally, the flour is blended through the creamed mixture, yielding a soft dough that lacks significant gluten formation because it is difficult for the flour proteins to gain access to the water they need for hydration. Short-dough biscuits are usually shaped by pressing the soft-dough into a mould cut into the metal roll of a rotary moulder (Manley 2000). After extraction from the mould, the pieces move quickly to the oven for baking.

Wire-cut cookies are also based on a relatively soft dough consistency with limited water content and gluten formation. In this case the individual pieces are formed by forcing the soft dough through a cylinder, or tube, and as it emerges from the end a wire, or knife, passes through the dough to cut off a unit piece of relevant size. This technique is particularly useful in the manufacture of cookies which contain particulate materials, like nuts and chocolate chips.

Hard-dough, semi-sweet biscuits require a greater degree of gluten formation and so added water levels tend to be a little higher (typically 20–25% flour weight), and fat and sugar levels somewhat lower. An all-in mixing process tends to be used, though multi-stage mixing methods are known. Modification of the dough rheological character may also be undertaken through the addition of a reducing agent, commonly sodium metabisulphite (Oliver et al. 1995), or a suitable source of proteolytic enzymes, or inactivated yeast. If it is not possible to modify the dough rheological properties through the addition of a reducing agent, extra water may be used to give a softer, more machinable dough. Hard-dough biscuits are usually made by sheeting the dough and then passing the sheet under a cutter, or series of cutters, to deliver the final biscuit shape for baking.

The degree of gluten formation in the manufacture of crackers needs to be greater than that with other biscuits to maintain the integrity of the dough and contribute to product lift. This means that dough water levels tend to be higher than with the biscuit types discussed above, but fat levels are lower. The mixing method used may deliberately set out to encourage gluten formation, though not to the same degree as achieved with bread dough. Crackers and some other biscuit forms, are made by sheeting the dough through pairs of smooth rolls, folding the sheet to create one or more layers (laminating), with further sheeting to reduce the thickness of the paste by passing through more rolls (Manley 2000). Fat or a fat-flour dust may be incorporated between the dough layers in order to increase the 'flakiness' of the product and there may be more than one laminating step. After the final sheeting reduction, the dough sheet passes under a cutter and the individual dough pieces are removed for baking.

Wafers are low fat biscuits produced from a batter. Water levels in the recipe are very high and the viscosity of the mix is sufficiently low to allow the batter to be deposited onto hot plates for baking. After depositing, a second plate is placed over the top of the one which holds the deposit and the pressure created from the heat of the oven and the restricting effect of the plates, forces the batter deposit to form a sheet of pre-determined thickness. Some deposited forms of biscuit are baked directly onto a hot plate and because of their high sugar content may remain flexible enough immediately after baking to be folded and shaped.

2.5 A Synopsis of Pastry Types and Manufacturing Processes

Short-dough pastes are used in a variety of bakery applications and products. The main forms can be classified according to whether they are used for the production of sweet or savoury products and are most commonly determined by whether sugar is present in the paste formulation, or not (Cauvain and Young 2006a). The other main form of pastry is commonly referred to as laminated pastry and includes puff pastry and yeasted examples such as croissant and Danish pastries. Laminated pastries may be sweetened or unsweetened. Pastry products are not often eaten alone but generally form part of a composite product, e.g. fruit pies. Significant gluten formation is not normally required in short-pastry products and if it occurs, may lead to problems during processing and baking. However, a reasonable degree of gluten formation is required in laminated pastries in order for the paste to withstand the considerable processing that is required to make laminated products. To meet the needs of this wide range of products, an equally wide range of mixing methods has been evolved.

As with biscuits, added water levels in paste formulations are kept to a minimum because much of the water is baked out in the oven to give a crisp eating character to the final baked pastry. Mixing methods for short-pastes may be all-in or multistage and in all cases, the aim is to limit gluten formation. The three multistage methods in common use for short-pastry production are:

- *Rubbing-in,* in which the flour and the fat are first mixed together before the addition of the water and soluble materials.
- *Creaming,* in which only half the fat and the flour are mixed together, followed by the addition of the remaining fat, water, and soluble materials (e.g. salt and sugars).
- *Boiling water,* in which the water (and sometimes the fat) is heated before being mixed with the other ingredients. This method is commonly used in the production of savoury pastes in the manufacture of meat pies.

After mixing, the short paste may be rested for a short period of time in order to modify the rheological properties of the paste and limit the risk of shrinkage. Short paste products are usually made by cutting shapes from a sheet of the paste and then forming into the required final shape. A particular means of forming base for short pastry products is by a process known as 'blocking', in which a small portion of the bulk paste (the 'billet') is placed in a foil or metal pan held in a shaped die and subjected to pressure from a second die moving downwards. The force of the downward moving die squeezes the paste into the narrow gap which is formed between the moving and static dies; the moving die is then withdrawn upwards and a paste shell remains behind ready for removal, filling with suitable sweet or savoury filling and then baking. Sometimes a sheeted (or rotary moulded) paste lid may be placed on the top of the filled product.

The procedures used in the manufacture of laminated pastes are very different. Laminated products tend to have a distinctive flaky eating character which is achieved by creating alternate layers of paste and fat (Cauvain and Young 2006a). Little fat is added to the base paste formulation and so gluten development is more likely to occur during mixing. Usually the gluten structure in the base dough is less well-developed than that in bread dough, because there is significant energy transfer to the paste during subsequent processing which adds to the gluten development that has occurred during mixing. The key rheological character of the base dough is such that it should be easily formed into a continuous sheet onto which the laminating fat is placed. A series of sheeting (thickness reduction) and folding (laminating) operations follows and this progressively builds up alternate and discrete layers of dough and fat. Resting stages may be used to modify the rheological properties of the paste, depending on the flour qualities and the product requirements. After sheeting and forming, un-yeasted laminated products (e.g. puff pastry) usually pass quickly to the oven, while yeasted laminated products will require a period of proof before they are ready for baking (*BakeTran* 2017a).

2.6 A Synopsis of Cake and Sponge Types and Manufacturing Processes

Cake batters are a complex emulsion and foam system (Cauvain 2003a; Cauvain and Young 2006a). In their simplest form, cake batters comprise wheat flour, sugar, and whole egg. At the start of the batter mixing process, the egg and sugar are usually whisked together. The sugar goes into solution in the water present in the egg and large numbers of minute air bubbles are trapped in the batter by the surface-active proteins in the egg. These proteins form a protective film around the air bubbles, preventing them from coalescing and escaping from the batter. After air incorporation, the flour is added with a minimum of mixing to avoid destabilising the egg foam which has already been formed. Many cake recipes contain a proportion of oil or fats to improve both the initial eating quality (tenderness) of cakes and to reduce the loss of desired soft-eating qualities during storage. The addition of an oil or solid fat to a cake recipe changes the batter to an oil- (fat-) in-water emulsion, where the aqueous, continuous phase contains the dissolved sugars, hydrated proteins and suspended flour, and other ingredient particles. Adding an oil or fat to the recipe considerably reduces the foam-stabilising properties of the egg, and the main aeration mechanism now involves the fat, or the addition of some other suitable foam stabilising material, e.g. glycerol monostearate (Cauvain and Cyster 1996; Sahi 1999). The role of individual ingredients in cake formulations is particularly important in delivering the required final form, eating qualities (*BakeTran* 2012). Cake products tend to have an intermediate moisture content which makes them susceptible to mould growth and as discussed below, the control of product water activity is important in delivering safe products with an acceptable mould-free shelf-life (Cauvain and Young 2008).

In practice a number of complex mixing procedures have evolved to form cake batters (Cauvain 2003b). For example, the 'sugar-batter' process in which the initial mixing step is the creaming of the fat and sugar, with the aim of aiding air incorporation before the addition of other ingredients, and the 'flour-batter' process, in which part of the flour and the fat are creamed together to aid air incorporation and limit gluten formation (Cauvain and Young 2006a). In many cases the need for elaborate multistage mixing processes was based on the use of ingredients in their 'traditional' form, e.g. milk, or to compensate for significant variations in ingredient character, e.g. butter composition. Today, provided that sufficient water is available to dissolve and hydrate the necessary ingredients, many cake batters can be based on a single-stage, all-in mixing method and little advantage will be gained from the more complex multistage methods. However, changes in the levels of key functional ingredients (such as may occur when developing nutritionally enhanced bakery products) may well require the use of more complicated multistage mixing methods.

Cake batters are low viscosity systems by comparison with bread and biscuit doughs and there is limited opportunity for a gluten structure to develop during mixing; in part because of the low resistance of the batter to the action of the mixer and in part, because of the gluten-inhibitory effects of sugar and fat in the recipe. The low viscosity of the batter after mixing makes it easy to deposit individual portions of batter into containers for subsequent baking. A few cake products are baked based on highly aerated sponge recipes (e.g. Swiss roll) and are deposited directly onto the oven band, or onto trays in thin sheets for rapid baking. In such products the tendency for the batter to flow is quickly restricted by the oven heat.

The characteristic eating qualities of cakes are significantly influenced by the level of batter aeration during mixing, the retention of that air which has been incorporated, and the thermal gas expansion and generation of steam during baking. As discussed briefly above the role of gas retention in cake batters is mainly the responsibility of the egg proteins, the fat and any emulsifiers that are present, rather than the gluten-forming proteins in the flour. Chemical aeration through the addition of a suitable baking powder (combination of food acid and sodium bicarbonate) in the recipe usually augments the mechanical aeration which comes from mixing (*BakeTran* 2017b).

2.7 The Key Sensory Properties of Bakery Products

While the sensory properties of bakery products vary widely from soft and moist to hard and brittle, they are dominated by two major inputs; their structure (texture) and moisture content. The texture of the different groups of products result in part, from the initial recipe formulation but perhaps more importantly, by the manner in which various structures are formed by the processing methods employed. As an important recipe ingredient, water plays major roles in structure formation, but perhaps the major impact of water content is more closely associated with the final moisture content of the product (Cauvain and Young 2008). The key role for water in determining the shelf-life of bakery products is considered below.

It is necessary to consider the key sensory properties which characterise bakery products, since these comprise major elements in the acceptance of bakery products by consumers and such properties are entrenched in consumer expectations of product quality and are 'sensed' even before a product is consumed. Thus, the delivery of nutritionally enhanced bakery products must take into account such consumer expectations. It is particularly important to recognise and understand the importance of product structure, since changes in texture can have significant impacts on product flavour, another sensory property important in meeting customer expectations (as discussed below).

In the consideration of the underlying technology used to manufacture bakery products above, some of the important attributes for the different sub-groups of bakery products have been introduced. They have been summarised for biscuits, crackers and cookies in Table 2.1 and are expanded and further considered for other bakery product sub-groups in Table 2.2. It should be noted that for each of the sub-groups identified, there will be significant regional variations in the final product texture and flavour. Such variations will mostly have an historical basis. This can be particularly true when it comes to the

Table 2.2 Important characteristics of bakery product sub-groups.

Product sub-group	Key technology	Range of textures	Product examples	Flavour	Moisture content
Bread	Gluten development and fermentation	Crust: from soft to hard and brittle Crumb: aerated, soft, resilient, slightly chewy	Crust: Pan sandwich to baguette Crumb: Pan sandwich to ciabatta	Neutral to slightly sour	Crust: 12–15% Crumb: 35–42%
Buns and rolls	Gluten development and fermentation	Crust: from soft to hard and brittle Crumb: aerated, soft, resilient, slightly chewy	Crust: hamburger buns to crusty rolls Crumb: aerated, soft, resilient, slightly chewy	Slightly sweet to slightly sour	Crust: 12–15% Crumb: 35–45%
Plain cakes	No gluten formation	Crust: soft Crumb: aerated and soft, limited resilience	All plain types	Sweet	22–28%
Fruited cakes	No gluten formation	Crust: soft Crumb: slightly dense and slightly firm	All fruited types	Sweet and fruity	20–28%
Savoury short pastry	Limited gluten formation combined with low recipe water content and fat	Crisp	Meat pie	Neutral	Crisp pastry 12–18%
Sweet short pastry	Limited gluten formation combined with low recipe water content, inclusion of and fat and sugar	Crisp	Fruit pies	Sweet	Crisp pastry 12–18%

Puff and Danish pastries, croissant	Modest gluten formation, fermentation (not puff pastry), combined with high recipe fat, sugar, sheeting, and lamination	Crisp and flaky	All types	From neutral to sweet	3–8%
Crackers and other laminated biscuits	Modest gluten formation (possibly with fermentation for crackers) combined with high recipe fat, sheeting, and lamination	Brittle and flaky		Neutral to slightly sweet	3–5%
Semi-sweet	Limited gluten formation combined with low recipe water, inclusion of fat and sugar and sheeting	Hard		Slightly sweet	3–5%
Short dough	No gluten formation combined with low recipe water, inclusion of fat and sugar	Short		Sweet	3–5%

(*Continued*)

Table 2.2 (Continued)

Product sub-group	Key technology	Range of textures	Product examples	Flavour	Moisture content
Cookies	No gluten formation combined with low recipe water, inclusion of fat and sugar	Short and tender		Sweet	3–5%
Wafers	No gluten formation combined with higher recipe water content and sugar	Short and brittle		Slightly sweet	3–5%

subject of bakery product sweetness, as illustrated by the examples for sugar levels in the bread recipes considered in Table 2.3.

As summarised in Table 2.2 (and discussed above), bread and other fermented products are characterised by having an aerated, cellular structure in the crumb of the final product which confers both softness and resilience to the crumb, along with a degree of chewiness. The foundation of this character is the development of a strong gluten network in the dough, which significantly contributes to the aerated character by first trapping air during mixing and then carbon dioxide gas from yeast fermentation. The additions of fats and sugars has a restricting effect on gluten formation, but because the levels of addition are modest, the overall effect is usually small and the bread crumb retains a degree of chewiness. The high moisture content of bread crumb is a significant contributor to its softness and the lower moisture content of bread crust is a significant contributor to crumb hardness or crispness.

Almost all types of cake are characterised by having an aerated, cellular crumb structure, though the degree of aeration is less than that of breads, not least because there is limited formation of a gluten structure. While cakes are more dense and their moisture contents lower than that of breads, their eating character remains soft because of higher levels of recipe fats and sugars. Most pastry and biscuit products are characterised by having the lowest moisture contents of all bakery products. Their low moisture contents are in part, the result of lower recipe water levels which, combined with the processing of the pastes and shapes into thin sheets, results in there being little residual moisture in the baked product. Such products are therefore characterised by hard and brittle textures, often modified through the introduction of recipe fat by varying process technologies (see above) which delivers a less brittle eating character.

2.8 Shelf-Life of Bakery Products

The shelf-life of bakery products can be described in two ways; as microbial-free or by changes in sensory qualities. The microbial-free shelf-life of bakery products is largely determined by the product Equilibrium Relative Humidity (ERH) or water activity (a_w). The reader is referred elsewhere for a more detailed consideration of the factors which impact the microbial-free shelf-life of bakery products

Table 2.3 Nutritional profiles of some common bakery products (100 g baked weight).

Product	Salt[a]	Fat	Saturated fat	Sugar	Dietary fibre	Protein	Energy (kcal)
White bread	1.0–1.7	2.0–3.0	0.4–1.0	1.5–4.0	2.0–3.0	8.0–10.0	265–280
Wholemeal bread	0.4–0.8	2.5–3.0	0.4–1.0	1.8–4.0	2.8–6.0	8.0–9.0	~280
Bread with seeds	~1.3	~3.5	~0.4	~2.0	~2.7	~8.0	~280
White hamburger buns	0.8–1.0	3–8	1.5–3	3–10	2–5	9–12	~260
Plain cake[b]	0.5–0.6	10–20	5–8	25–40	0.8–1.2	5–8	~350
Blueberry muffins	~1.25	~13.5	~1.0	~25.0	~1.5	~4.1	~335
Fruited cake	0.2–0.4	8–10	4–6	35–45	2–4	4–6	~350
Cookies	0.8–1.0	12–20	0–10	10–30	2–5	6–10	~400
Croissant (plain)	0.7–0.8	15–20	8–12	5–8	2–4	8–10	~380
Crumpets[c]	~1.5	~2.0	~0.5	~2.0	~1.7	~9.5	~210
Jam doughnut[d]	~1.3	~11.0	~5.0	~10.0	~2.0	~5.5	~320

NB: nutritional profiles will vary widely in products sub-groups and in geographical regions. The values quoted are provided are to put into context the discussions which follow. The data are only indicative; they have been gathered and summarised by the authors based on a selection of pack declarations.

[a] Sodium converted to salt (sodium chloride) equivalents; salt = sodium × 2.5.

[b] No top icing or cream filling.

[c] Product baked on a hot-plate.

[d] Includes jam filling.

(e.g. Cauvain and Young 2008). Particularly important in the context of the subject of this work, is the recognition of the key roles played by two ingredients, salt and sugar, in determining the microbial-free shelf-life of bakery products and in many cases, product safety for the consumer. With a recognition of the importance of their roles in determining the microbial-free shelf-life of bakery products, must come an understanding that product reformulation involving these ingredients predicates a need to take other relevant measures related to food safety. As will be discussed in relevant sections below, the latter is not a trivial task, and may require significant and far-reaching changes of the manufacture of consumer-acceptable nutritionally enhanced bakery products. It is important to recognise that product moisture makes a number of very important contributions to final product character. Firstly, product moisture content is a major contributor to and related to, product ERH (and therefore microbial-free shelf-life). However, there are many other recipe components which influence ERH and product moisture content alone cannot be used as the sole determinant of the microbial-free shelf-life of a bakery product.

The second key role for moisture is in contributing to the overall eating qualities of different bakery products. Again, the nature of the contribution depends on the particular sub-class of bakery products being considered. For most cakes and bread crumb, the higher the moisture content the softer will be the product, which is important because consumers of such products commonly equate product softness with 'freshness'. For bread products the role of moisture is complex. With some bread products, such as baguettes, consumer expectations are for a crisp (hard) crust, which would not be the case with higher moisture contents. For other bread products, such as sandwich breads and hamburger buns, the expectation is for a soft crust. For the majority of pastry and biscuit products, consumers associate low moisture contents with acceptable product quality and higher moisture contents would not be seen as a 'normal' characteristics for such products.

The eating character and to some extent the flavour, of bakery products changes in storage post-baking. The nature of the changes is complex and varies with the particular sub-group being considered. These post-baking changes are commonly called staling, though the interpretation of the concept as to what constitutes a 'stale' product (i.e. one which has unacceptable eating characteristics) varies with the product. Some changes in post-baking product character are associated with moisture loss from, absorption by, or moisture movement within the product; with the latter being possible at the macro level (e.g. crumb to crust, or product to atmosphere), or at the micro level (e.g. starch to protein, or vice versa). Essentially, many consumers see staling as a loss of a range of desirable product characteristics which they commonly associate with freshness. In this context, there can be a distinct difference in consumer perceptions of product quality depending on how and when, they purchase products. Purchases from a local bakery are commonly assumed to be fresh, since the product may be warm and the environment indicative of baking activity, e.g. the smell of baking. In contrast, products purchased in larger retail environments are often divorced from intimate baking operations, in that they will be cold and wrapped. Such differences have to be taken into account when considering recipe and process changes which impact on staling, not least because a number of common bakery ingredients contribute anti-staling effects.

As already noted, the concept of staling varies with bakery products. In the case of pastries and biscuits, staling is most commonly associated with the absorption of water by the product with the subsequent loss of crispness. In contrast with cakes and bread it is the loss of water causing the products to become hard that is associated with staling. However, even when cakes and bread are wrapped in a moisture impermeable film to prevent moisture loss, cakes and especially bread, will continue to lose their softness with increased storage time. This change is brought about by changes at the micro (molecular) level and are associated with the physical state of proteins and starch. The reader is referred elsewhere for a more detailed discussion of such changes (e.g. Cauvain and Young 2008; Rayas-Duarte and Mulvaney 2012).

2.9 Nutritional Profiles of Common Bakery Products

The nutritional profiles of bakery products vary widely, in part based on the ratios of recipe ingredients which have evolved over many years and which have become synonymous with the character of the various product sub-groups. In addition, there are geographical variations associated with a given bakery product; an example of such geographical variation has already been introduced for bread in Table 2.3. The differences in the major nutritional profiles for some common bakery products are also illustrated in Table 2.3 to allow the reader to appreciate some 'typical' starting points for the development of nutritionally enhanced bakery products; more detailed considerations are presented below in the discussion of the opportunities for new product development and relevant approaches to development examples. The data presented are derived from generic published recipes and the focus is on the major nutritional components.

As already illustrated by Cauvain and Young (2006b), biscuits, cookies and crackers in Europe are higher in recipe fat and sugar levels than breads and many fermented products which means that they are more energy dense per 100 g. In addition, Table 2.3 shows that such products are lower in dietary fibre. However, while the analytical data may highlight nutritional differences between products, due account must be taken with respect to common levels of consumption of biscuits compared with bread products. Cake products tend to have the highest levels of recipe fat and sugar, and lowest fibre levels of all baked products, but are perhaps less regularly consumed and are often viewed by consumers as indulgent products.

The challenges and opportunities for the development of nutritionally enhanced bakery products will be discussed in detail below, but based on the nutritional data presented in Table 2.3 they may be summarised as:

- Reductions in recipe salt levels.
- Increases in dietary fibre.
- Reductions in recipe sugars.
- Reductions in total recipe fat.
- Reductions in recipe saturated fats.
- Reductions in energy density.

From the preceding discussion, it is clear that the degree of nutritional enhancement which may be achieved will vary according to the under-pinning technology used for the manufacture of bakery product sub-groups and as noted earlier, geographical location. For example, in many cases bread is made without the addition of recipe sugar, with the analytical data reflecting the levels of naturally occurring sugars in wheat flour, in some cases being in total as high as 3% (MacArthur and D'Appolonia 1979).

Given this level of naturally occurring sugars, the opportunities for sugar reduction in many bread products appears limited, with the exception of those parts of the world where non-wheat flour sugars are added to the bread recipe (see examples in Table 2.3). While bread is seen as a suitable vehicle for delivering higher dietary fibre levels (e.g. via wholemeal or bran-enriched breads), the potentially negative effects of dietary-rich materials on the texture and taste of cakes and pastries may limit their acceptance by consumers.

2.10 Conclusion

The term 'bakery' covers a range of food products with diverse textures and tastes, formed as the result of complex ingredient–recipe–process interactions. Almost all bakery products are based on wheat with the formation, or not, of a gluten network in the product matrix being a significant factor in determining the final product structure. Fat and sugar are two recipe ingredients which make major contributions to final product structure and eating qualities, and while reduction in their levels may be desirable nutritionally, undoubtedly there will be major quality changes which will have to be overcome in order to deliver consumer-acceptable products. Water not only plays major roles in the manufacture of the different sub-groups of bakery products, but also makes major contributions to product texture and shelf-life, both sensory and microbial. Particular processing technologies have been evolved to deal with the manufacture of the different sub-groups of bakery products and in this context the roles of ingredient salt, fat, and sugar are important.

It is clear that 'simple' reduction of one recipe ingredient to nutritionally enhance a particular product may have other negative effects on the nutritional composition of the final product. In addition, a single ingredient change can have major implications for product preparation, processing, and final product quality. Thus, the delivery of nutritionally enhanced bakery products requires a thorough understanding of the under-pinning product technology, and a recognition that processing changes may be required in order to deliver suitable and acceptable final products to consumers.

References

BakeTran (2012). A guide to the main effects of the main ingredients used in cake and sponge recipes. In: *Chorleywood Bookshelf Monograph Series*, vol. 3. Witney, UK: (www.baketran.com).

BakeTran (2017a). Technology of laminated products. In: *Chorleywood Bookshelf Monograph Series*, vol. 4. Witney, UK: (www.baketran.com).

BakeTran (2017b). A guide to chemical leavening agents and baking powders, and their application on baked products. In: *Chorleywood Bookshelf Monograph Series*, vol. 5. Witney, UK: (www.baketran.com).

Calvel, R., Wirtz, R.L., and MacGuire, J.J. (2001). *The Taste of Bread*. Gaithersburg, MA: Aspern Publishers Inc.

Campbell, G.M. and Martin, P.J. (2012). Bread aeration and dough rheology: an introduction. In: *Breadmaking: Improving Quality*, 2e (ed. S.P. Cauvain), 299–336. Cambridge, UK: Woodhead Publishing.

Cauvain, S.P. (1994). New mixer for variety bread production. European Food and Drink Review (Autumn): 51–53.

Cauvain, S.P. (2001). Breadmaking. In: *Cereal Processing Technology* (ed. G. Owens), 204–230. Cambridge, UK: Woodhead Publishing.

Cauvain, S.P. (2003a). Nature of cakes. In: *Encyclopaedia of Food Science and Nutrition*, 2e (ed. B. Caballero, L. Trogo and P.M. Finglas), 751–756. St Louis, MO:: Academic Press.

Cauvain, S.P. (2003b). Methods of manufacture. In: *Encyclopaedia of Food Science and Nutrition*, 2e (ed. B. Caballero, L. Trogo and P.M. Finglas), 756–759. St Louis, MO: Academic Press.

Cauvain, S.P. (2015). *Technology of Breadmaking*, 3e. Cham, Switzerland: Springer International Publishing AG.

Cauvain, S.P. (2016a). Sour dough technology. In: *Encyclopedia of Food Grains*, 2e (ed. C. Wrigley, H. Corke, K. Seetharaman and J. Faubion)), 25–29. Oxford: Academic Press.

Cauvain, S.P. (2016b). Cookies, biscuits and crackers: formulation, processing and characteristics. In: *Encyclopedia of Food Grains*, 2e (ed. C. Wrigley, H. Corke, K. Seetharaman and J. Faubion), 37–43. Oxford: Academic Press.

Cauvain, S.P. and Cyster, J.A. (1996) Sponge cake technology. *CCFRA Review No. 2*. Chipping Campden, UK: Campden BRI.

Cauvain, S.P. and Young, L.S. (2006a). *Baked Products: Science, Technology and Practice*. Oxford, UK:: Blackwell Publishing.

Cauvain, S.P. and Young, L.S. (2006b). *The Chorleywood Bread Process*. Cambridge, UK: Woodhead Publishing.

Cauvain, S.P. and Young, L.S. (2008). *Bakery Food Manufacture and Quality: Water Control and Effects*, 2e. Oxford, UK: Wiley-Blackwell.

Cauvain, S.P., Cato, L., and Ma, J. (2015). A review of some aspects of the practical importance of assessing flour quality and dough rheology in the manufacture of bread and laminated pastries. Cereal Technology (March): 28–137.

Dobraszczyk, B.J., Campbell, G.M., and Gan, Z. (2001). Bread: a unique food. In: *Cereals and Cereal Products* (ed. D.A.V. Dendy and B.J. Dobraszczyk), 182–232. Gaithersburg, MA: Aspen Publishers.

Gobbetti, M. and Ganzle, M. (2013). *Handbook on Sourdough Technology*. New York, NY: Springer Science+Business Media.

Huang, S. (2014). Steamed bread. In: *Bakery Products Science and Technology*, 2e (ed. W. Zhou), 539–562. Oxford, UK: Wiley Blackwell.

MacArthur, L.A. and D'Appolonia, B.L. (1979). Comparison of oat and wheat carbohydrates, 1. Sugars. Cereal Chemistry 56: 455–457.

Manley, D. (2000). *Technology of Biscuits, Crackers and Cookies*, 3e. Cambridge, UK:: Woodhead Publishing.

Oliver, G., Thacker, D., and Wheeler, R.J. (1995). Semi-sweet biscuits: 1. The influence of sodium metabisulphite on dough rheology and baking performance. Journal of the Science of Food and Agriculture 69: 141–150.

Rayas-Duarte, P. and Mulvaney, S. (2012). Bread staling. In: *Breadmaking: Improving Quality*, 2e (ed. S.P. Cauvain), 580–596. Cambridge, UK: Woodhead Publishing.

Sahi, S.S. (1999). Influence of aeration and emulsifiers on cake batter rheology and textural properties of cake. In: *Bubbles in Food* (ed. G.M. Campbell, C. Webb, S.S. Pandiella and K. Niranjan), 263–271. St. Paul, MN: AACC.

Schunemann, C. and Treu, G. (2001). *Baking; the Art and Science*, 2e. Calgary, Canada: Baker Tech Inc.

Wilde, P. (2012). Foam formation in dough and bread quality. In: *Breadmaking: Improving Quality*, 2e (ed. S.P. Cauvain), 337–351. Cambridge, UK: Woodhead Publishing.

3

Delivering Health Benefits via Bakery Products

3.1 Micronutrients

No single food is capable of delivering all of the health benefits required in the human diet. In all countries throughout the world, diets comprise a mixture of food sources and thus offer the potential for delivering a balanced diet. There is the need for access to sufficient total energy based on a variety of individual energy sources, e.g. fat, protein and carbohydrates. The position of these dietary sources with respect to human health and bakery products will be discussed in subsequent chapters. In addition to the major dietary sources of energy, there are many other nutrients which play significant roles in human health, even though they are consumed at much lower levels than the major energy sources. Such nutrients are commonly referred to as 'micronutrients' and are usually required in the human diet in small quantities. In some cases, excess consumption of these 'trace elements' may lead to negative health benefits and even toxic effects. The need for micronutrients in a healthy human diet has long been recognised, as exemplified by the historical references to the use of lime juice to obviate the effects of scurvy for British sailors in the eighteenth century (eventually giving rise to the North American slang term 'Limeys' when referring to British sailors).

The two main groups of micronutrients can be considered under the headings of vitamins and minerals. While the quantity of micronutrients can be readily measured analytically, this does not present the true position with regard to their effectiveness in the diet. The true measure of the value of a micronutrient lies with its bioavailability, that is, how

Baking Technology and Nutrition: Towards a Healthier World, First Edition.
Stanley P. Cauvain and Rosie H. Clark.

it will be active and available during the processes of digestion and its ability to be absorbed in the human intestinal system. In this respect the role of the micronutrients is complex and knowledge of the processes involved is continually evolving as nutritional research progresses. Within this complex context, the addition of micronutrients to bakery foods and any associated claims need to be carefully weighed in the development of nutritionally enhanced bakery products.

Cereal grains are considered to be a useful source of micronutrients in the diet. However, the milling of grains, such as wheat to provide a 'refined' product (white flour) for use in the manufacture of many baked products, may have a potentially negative impact on the overall nutritive value of the resultant flour. The proportion of the wheat grain converted to flour is commonly referred to by the term 'extraction rate' (Owens 2001). An extraction rate of 100% indicates that all of the wheat has been converted to flour, so that anything less than 100% indicates that a proportion of bran (and germ) have been removed. In flours with less than 100% extraction, the endosperm component of the wheat grain will dominate. White flour extraction rates vary, and commonly range from 65% to 75%. The extraction rate of wheat flour is commonly associated with the analytical measurement of ash (Cauvain 2018), as the branny layers of wheat are rich in minerals. Thus, a low ash value (<0.5%) would indicate a low level of branny materials in the white flour, with higher ash levels being associated with higher extraction rates. The relationship between wheat flour ash and extraction rate is not straightforward as it depends on the way in which the milling procedures are set up. Dewettinck et al. (2008) provided a comprehensive review of the chemical composition of wheat flours with different extractions rates. Their data confirm the important contribution that the branny layers make to the vitamin and mineral content of the final flour and confirm that lower levels of both types of micronutrient remain after processing wheat grains to white flour.

3.2 Vitamins and Antioxidants

The compounds that we call vitamins fall into two broad categories, those which are fat soluble (A, D, E, and K) and those which are water soluble (C and B-group). The naming of vitamins, for historical reasons, is not straightforward (Wagner and Folkers 1964). In addition to the commonly used nomenclature, vitamins may also be described by their chemical names. For example, vitamin C is often described as ascorbic acid and even has an E-number, E 300. Ascorbic acid is a common component of bread improvers around the world; though in this role it is not being used for nutritional reasons but for its technological function in the oxidation of wheat flour proteins during the formation of gluten (Cauvain 2015).

Vitamins can be sourced directly from many foods and are required in small amounts in the diet of humans. About 12 vitamins are required for a healthy metabolism in the human body. A particular problem with some vitamins (for example the vitamin B-group and vitamin C) is that they are not completely stable during food processing, including cooking and baking (Burch 2011). This can mean that while vitamin supplementation of raw materials or product recipes and formulations may be practised, the level of vitamins remaining in a finished baked product may be lower than that of the starting formulae. Because of such losses the likelihood for passing the full nutritional benefits of vitamin supplements to consumers in baked products may be reduced. In some cases, the effectiveness of vitamins may be enhanced when consumed with other micronutrients.

In addition to the potential impact of the heat input during baking in lowering the value of vitamin levels in baked products, a significant barrier to improving the vitamin contribution of baked goods is that many of the natural sources of the relevant vitamins are associated with raw materials not commonly used as ingredients in bakery foods recipes, for example vegetables. The B-group vitamins are present in whole grains though, because of their concentration in the bran and germ (embryo) of cereals, the processing of grains to yield white flour does lead to a potential reduction of their contribution to the diet. In some cases (see above and below), this depletion of B-group vitamins from the processing of grains has led to the mandatory and voluntary fortification of white flours destined for the manufacture of baked products. In 2014, the European Food Safety Authority (EFSA 2014) published an opinion on the safety of vitamin D-enriched UV-treated bakers' yeast, which has led to its common use for the manufacture of bread through in-store bakeries in the UK (Anon 2014). Vitamin D is important for maintaining the calcium balance in the body and is therefore important in the formation and maintenance of a healthy bone structure. Exposure to sunlight boosts the vitamin D levels in the body, but large numbers of consumers live in parts of the world where exposure to sunlight may be limited and thus, the promise was that delivery of vitamin D via fortified yeast would have potential benefits for many individuals. Other recent developments have shown that is possible to develop grains which may make more significant vitamin contributions to the diet. For example, rice has been developed which delivers high levels of *beta*-carotene (vitamin A in its carotenoid form) which can aid in combatting blindness and improving the overall nutrition in geographical areas where rice forms the major portion of the human diet. Commonly known as the 'Golden rice project', the product relied on the genetic manipulation of rice grains to deliver specific health benefits and because of that has not met with universal approval or acceptance.

Cereals are a source of antioxidants, phytochemicals (Slavin et al. 2001) and phytoestrogens of the lignin family (Adlercreutz and Mazur 1997). These are compounds which are linked with potentially beneficial effects in slowing down the ageing process (which results from oxidative damage to DNA), and a possible protective effect against some hormone-related cancers in adults. Antioxidants are also associated with an ability to limit the deterioration of foods, including the rancidity of fatty acids and discolouration (Young and O'Sullivan 2011). The term antioxidant covers a wide range of substances including some enzymes, phenolics, flavonoids, and some complementary agents (e.g. vitamin C) (Hegarty 1992). In the context of baking, the appearance of vitamin C (ascorbic acid) may seem adventitious, but it is worth remembering that the processes involved with baking do not necessarily guarantee the survival of the ascorbic acid to take part in antioxidant activity post-baking.[1] The antioxidant role of ascorbic acid in the manufacture of baked products may be seen through its effect on reducing the discolouration of apple slices used for fruit pies and less commonly, through its addition to potato pieces if they are required to stand for any length of time in the manufacture of savoury pies.

1 Readers are reminded that while ascorbic acid is commonly referred to chemically as an antioxidant or reduced agent, bakers commonly refer to it as an 'oxidant', since in breadmaking the interaction of ascorbic acid with atmospheric oxygen in the presence of the ascorbate enzyme in wheat flour, converts it to dehydro-ascorbic acid which acts as the oxidising agent on the gluten-forming proteins (Cauvain 2015).

3.3 Minerals

Minerals are inorganic materials which are involved in the healthy functioning of the human body. They occur at low (trace) levels in many different raw materials and are stored in plants through absorption from the soil while they are growing. Thus, the mineral content of the soil plays an important part in determining the mineral composition and the level of individual minerals which may be present in a raw material. Animal and seafood products also play a role in delivering essential minerals to the human diet. Because minerals are inorganic they are not destroyed during processing, but may be prone to leaching out into any process water used in the food preparation, particularly during soaking. The distribution of minerals throughout a plant matrix may not be uniform and it may be that processing depletion may occur in the preparation of different forms of a raw material. For example, many of the minerals in wheat and other grains are associated with the outer branny and aleurone layers. In the case of wheat, this means that white flour tends to have lower levels of minerals present than wholemeal flour, a fact which is involved with the process of flour fortification, as discussed above and below.

As is the case with vitamins, the food sources for many minerals involved in human nutrition are not commonly used in the manufacture of bakery products. Some common bakery related sources of minerals are listed in Table 3.1 and others are discussed in the section on flour fortification below. Table 3.1 shows that bakery products have the potential to deliver a wide spectrum of important dietary minerals, with wholegrains making particularly important contributions. The ability to make specific claims regarding the positive contribution of a bakery product to mineral-related health benefits is limited and highly regulated. In most cases, to meet a health-related claim it is most likely that the natural background level of a specific mineral would need to be supplemented; the approach to bakery raw materials fortification is further discussed below.

3.4 Fortification of Flour and Bakery Products

The delivery of health benefits to consumers via food systems has long been practised, not least through the principle of fortification of specified foods with nutrients in part, to improve the overall diet of

Table 3.1 Sources of minerals in common bakery raw materials.

Mineral	Bakery raw materials
Calcium	Milk and dairy products
Copper	Nuts
Chromium	Yeast
Fluoride	Fluoridated water
Magnesium	Nuts, sesame seeds, wheat
Manganese	Wholegrains, seeds, nuts, cocoa, yeast
Molybdenum	Wholegrains, milk products
Phosphorus	Skim milk, nuts, sesame, pumpkin, and sunflower seeds
Selenium	Brazil nuts, wholegrains wheat (especially germ), dairy products
Sodium	Cereal grains, salt, baking powders, dried fruits
Zinc	Wholegrains, nuts, soya beans, pecans, pumpkin, and sunflower seeds.

populations who are considered to be receiving sub-optimal nutrition and in part, to 'restore' nutrients which may be 'missing' as the result of the processing of raw materials into final products. The approaches used to convey nutritional guidelines to improve diet and health vary in detail around the world. In the case of wheat flour, fortification with specific nutrients, minerals, and vitamins is widely practised. The technical issues associated with fortification tend to be few and are more concerned with the processes associated with treating the flour, than with the production of the final baked product. Thus, while fortification will be considered as part of this work, it is not its main focus.

The most common applications of flour fortification have been, and still are, made with respect to the calcium, iron, and B vitamins. As noted above, early moves to fortification were related to the restriction of diets in times of conflict. More recently the same concerns have been related to the differences between wholemeal and white flours, with the latter being seen as 'deficient' in certain nutrients with respect to the former. While it is true that the mineral and vitamin content of white wheat flours are lower than those of wholemeal, this does not imply (as some commentators would state) that the consumption of white bread products does not make significant dietary contributions to human diets. The nutritional position regarding wholemeal versus white flour is complex. It is true that wholemeal flours are rich in dietary fibre, complex carbohydrates, B-vitamins, iron, and minerals in comparison with white flour, but they are also a source of phytic acid (in the bran). Phytic acid is known to be associated with hindering the absorption of some minerals (Davies and Nightingale 1975; Rosell 2012), thus reducing the potential effectiveness of wholemeal flour in nutrition terms. It is worth noting that there may be other potentially negative nutritional factors associated with wholemeal flours, including potential higher levels of mycotoxins. Schaarschmidt and Fauhl-Hassek (2018) provided a comprehensive review of the problems associated with mycotoxins in wheat and the potential for complying with the maximum legal limits being imposed by the EU. They concluded that for white bread, the practices involved could ensure compliance, while 'In the case of wholemeal products, bran-enriched products, or high-cereal low-moisture bakery products, this appears to be challenging and improved technology and/or selection of high-quality raw materials would be required'. In addition to the greater risk of the presence of mycotoxins, wholemeal flours have the practical problem of rancidity arising from the presence of the vitamin rich wheat germ during long-term storage; a factor noted in Chapter 1, which was an integral part of the development of the germ-enriched bread known as Hovis. Changes related to rancidity also contribute to the more rapid loss of baking performance of wholemeal flours during storage compared with white flours.

In more recent years there has been a move to fortify flours with folic acid. The primary rationale behind this particular aspect of flour fortification has been the reduction of the risk of child births with potential neural-tube defects, which could result in the development of medical conditions such as spina bifida. While the medical evidence has supported fortification (Department of Health 1992), there has not been a universal acceptance of the practice. In part the reluctance of some authorities has been associated with potential negative effects for sectors of the population suffering from vitamin B12 deficiency and epilepsy. In addition to the potentially ambiguous medical effects, the practical implications associated with product labelling and the added costs associated with fortification, have delayed the mandatory implementation of flour fortification in a number of parts of the world (including the UK). While there are strong imperatives for many, if not all, governments to improve the diet of a country's population, there can be equally strong imperatives for not doing so in those parts of the world where access to a varied diet at a reasonable cost is possible. In such cases there is less pressure for the mandatory fortification of foods.

3.5 Ancient Grains

In recent years interest has gradually emerged in 'so-called' ancient grains. Commonly this category includes wheats such as spelt, Kamut®, freekeh, farro, einkorn and emmer, along with other grains such as millet, barley, teff, oats and sorghum. The pseudo-cereals quinoa, amaranth, buckwheat, and chia, are also commonly considered in this context, and even wild rice, sprouted wheat and lupins. There is no formal definition of what comprises an ancient grain and often it is their association with the 'ancient' past that has attracted wide attention in dietary circles, not least with respect to 'improved' digestibility of the native starch. They have also been linked with conditions described as 'wheat-intolerance' (these conditions should not be confused with the well-defined and understood coeliac disease). Taylor and Awika (2017) provide a comprehensive review of gluten-free ancient grains not related to wheat. They considered that such grains were characterised by their ability to produce a crop in environmental conditions which were not favourable for the growth of wheat.

Ancient wheats are often described as wheat types which have not changed over a long period, often considered to be 100 years, or more. This most certainly contrasts with modern wheat varieties which have a relatively 'short life', of maybe 20 years. The drivers of developing new wheat varieties are most commonly, increased pest and disease resistance, agricultural advantages from increased yield and drought-tolerance, and the ability to deliver improved functionality in the manufacture of the various sub-groups of bakery products for which the flour is destined. Differences in the potential contribution to human health between 'ancient and modern' types are not clear. In part this is because of the natural variation which may be encountered arising from different genotypes, environmental conditions and agricultural practices, all of which may have an influence. Gil et al. (2011) discussed the mechanism by which wheat confers positive health benefits in the human digestive system. Amongst the physical and chemical attributes that they identified, were the amount and type of fibre, the quantity and quality of the phytochemicals, and the ratio of amylose to amylopectin in the starch.

Some nutritional studies do conclude that the consumption of ancient grains have positive health benefits for humans. For example, Sofi et al. (2013) carried out clinical trials with Khorsan wheat (Kamut) using 22 healthy subjects in a randomised trial, and suggested that their results indicated that a replacement diet with Kamut wheat flour and semolina used in pasta, bread crackers and biscuits, could be effective in reducing metabolic risk factors. Participants were not allowed to eat any other grains during the trial. Dinu et al. (2018) provided a comprehensive consideration of the biochemical and chemical implications for the use of ancient grains with data and observations drawn from many *in vitro, ex vivo,* animal, and immune toxicity studies. Drawing on data from the Healthgrain project (https://healthgrain.org) for fibre and phytochemicals composition, Dinu et al. (2018) found limited evidence for the significant health benefits between ancient and modern wheats; though the latter had the highest fibre level of the wheats studied. In the context of human nutrition they considered that '... given the limited number of human trials, it is not possible to definitively conclude that ancient wheat varieties are superior to all modern counterparts in reducing chronic health disease'.

Though not strictly based on an ancient grain, the manufacture of 'flourless' bread, which uses sprouted wheat has begun to create interest. The manufacture of such bread was reported as long ago as 1999 in Russia, with Antonov et al. (2005) describing 'Tonus' bread and making many claims for its potential health benefits for humans. Amongst the benefits that they described were higher levels of vitamins and minerals and a host of health-related claims. The principle associated with the value of using spouted wheat for the manufacture of bread is the action of enzymes during the spouting process which breaks down the wheat proteins and carbohydrates (starch) yielding a food with a low glycaemic index which makes the bread 'more digestible' than 'standard' breads. At the time of writing no supporting objective evidence for such claims have come to light.

3.6 Functional Foods

In the context of delivering consumer health and well-being to humans, the concept of functional foods has developed (Hasler 1998). Such foods are most commonly based on delivering bioactive components which are present naturally in raw materials to deliver specific health benefits in final product formulations. They should not be confused with the manipulation of product formulations to deliver improved nutrition (e.g. lower sugar or fat). It may be that new product developments can combine both the inclusion of bioactive materials and improved background nutrition. Such developments would address the concept of 'Food as Medicine' (Ehrnreich 2000), at least in the sense that the formulation has been designed to deliver specific health benefits. It would be difficult to argue without supporting medical evidence that the introduction of a specific bioactive compound would contribute to combatting a particular disease or illness. However, it may be less difficult to argue that the introduction of specific bioactive compounds can assist in alleviating the symptoms of some medical conditions. In this sense functional foods may be viewed in much the same way as homeopathic medicine, where there is a long-standing tradition of using naturally bioactive materials. Korhonen (2002) considered food reformulation alone was not enough to deliver health benefits and that it would often be necessary to develop and apply, innovative technologies in order to facilitate the manufacture of functional foods. To support his case, the author provided examples relevant to the manufacture of dairy products. As discussed below, a particular challenge with using bioactive materials in baking relates to the high temperatures and long oven residence times associated with the manufacture of bakery products. Such conditions can readily lead to the degradation of many ingredients and potentially the loss of the bioactivity of the raw material concerned, a significant factor when considering the use of a bioactive material in product development.

The term nutraceutical may also be encountered in discussions on nutrition, most commonly in North America. As is the case with functional foods, the concept of a nutraceutical is not clearly defined but commonly, it refers to a chemical in or added to a food which, while not in itself a nutrient, does confer potential beneficial effects with respect to nutrition. Such ingredients may unlock the potential of other nutrients in a composite food, or combine with a nutrient in such a way as to increase its bioavailability within the human digestive system. Another term which may be encountered in the literature is 'designer foods'. This and other non-defined descriptors tend to be derived within a marketing environment (Siro et al. 2008) and seldom have any legislative standing. One exception defined as early as 1991 in Japan, was for 'Foods for Specified Health Use (FOSHU)'; since then they have moved to a self-regulating code of practice related to specific health claims (Eve 2000).

3.7 Prebiotics and Probiotics

The role of human gut microflora in supporting health is a specialist subject outside of the scope of this work, however, it is relevant to consider both prebiotics and probiotics since they are often considered in the formulation of healthier foods. Prebiotics are more likely to be considered in a bakery context than probiotics as they comprise non-digestible oligosaccharides and are often described as functional foods. As such, oligosaccharides often assay as fibre and thus, may be related to the potential for specific health benefits and claims. The prebiotics include derivatives of the sugars fructose and galactose, and they support the growth of bifidobacteria in the human colon. It is generally considered that their presence changes and potentially improves, the functions of colonic microflora. Prebiotics have a plant origin and are found in vegetables and some fruits. Prebiotic-rich ingredients are not commonly used in baked products, though a number have been considered (Padma Ishwarya and Prabhasankar 2014). Rich sources of prebiotics include chicory, bananas, gum acacia, leeks, and onions. Inulin is a soluble polymer of fructose found in root vegetables, a good source being the Jerusalem artichoke. Inulin remains largely undigested in the human digestive system and functions as a prebiotic. Available in a powder form, it has been proposed for use in bakery products as a low calorie bulking agent (Codina and Bilan 2006). A summary of potential prebiotics is given in Table 3.2. While the use of prebiotics in foodstuffs is widely accepted, readers are advised to check the local legislation with respect to their acceptance, limitations of level and labelling requirements.

Probiotics are preparations of microbial cultures which are added to foods with the intention of impacting, or restoring the balance of human gut microflora. Since the cultures need to be 'live' to achieve

Table 3.2 Examples of prebiotics.

Potential prebiotic	Typical sources
Inulin	Chicory and Jerusalem artichoke
Fructooligosaccharides	Inulin
Short chain fructooligosaccharides	Fermentation of cane of beet sugar
Oligofructose	Enzymic hydrolysis of inulin
Isomalto-oligosaccharides	Processed starches
Polydextrose	Manufactured polymer of glucose
Resistant starch	Various starches
Resistant dextrins	Wheat, maize, and tapioca
Lactitol	Dairy derivative
Tagatose	Dairy products
Gum arabic	*Acacia* tree exudates
Partially hydrolysed guar gum	Guar plant seeds
Soya oligosaccharides	Soya beans and peas
Pyrodextrins	Mixtures of oligosaccharides

their functional objectives, they will be susceptible to the effects of heat and so tend not to have a significant role in baked products. There is the potential to encapsulate a probiotic to limit the adverse effects of processing, however, the nature of common encapsulating materials means that they are unlikely to cope sufficiently well with the harsh conditions in a bakery oven to be able to deliver a viable probiotic effect.

3.8 'Botanicals'

Botanical ingredients were first encountered in the context of cosmetic or personal care products. The term refers to materials which originate or are derived from plants, most commonly herbs, roots, flowers, fruits, leaves, or seeds. The use of the descriptor has become more widespread and now includes references to the inclusion of such ingredients in baked products, with the assumption that the use of such specific ingredients may bring or be associated with particular health benefits, not least because of their chemical structure. The application of the term to baked products is somewhat removed from the original usage of the term, not least because the use of 'botanical' agents in skin care products where they have not been subjected to the effects of oven baking is at best, misleading as to the practical benefits of their addition to baked products. Recipes for bakery products which use fruits, herbs, spices, and vegetable additions have been known for many years (David 1977; Davidson 1995; Shapter 1999). In some cases this has been the result of the need to dilute the proportion of wheat flour in a bakery product mix at times of nutritional stress for particular populations. Recipes for bakery products at times of global conflicts have often been adapted to include ingredients such as potatoes, tomatoes, and beetroot.

3.9 Allergens and Special Diets

Knowledge of allergic responses to certain raw materials and foods has increased significantly in recent years, so that their presence in a bakery food is clearly labelled and largely understood by consumers. Many allergens are responsible for immediate hypersensitivity reactions and cause symptoms which vary from mild to acute, and potentially life-threatening. The individual response to an allergen varies. Common allergies which may find their place in bakery products are those related to peanuts, tree nuts, egg, cow's milk, sesame seeds, and soya beans. In many cases it is possible to re-formulate bakery products to remove the offending allergen and to substitute another material to provide the necessary functionality in the baked product. The development of 'free-from' bakery products is increasing, with new versions regularly reaching the market. In some cases such allergen-free products are consumed as part of a lifestyle choice and not necessarily as the result of a known allergic reaction.

Coeliac disease (gluten-sensitive enteropathy) is probably the best known allergic response related to bakery products. This condition is very different to the allergic reactions noted above, and is a cell-mediated allergic reaction to the wheat storage protein known as gliadin, a major component of the many cereals, wheat especially. The reader is referred elsewhere for a detailed discussion of the condition (Troncone and Auricchio 1991) which is associated with inflammation of the epithelial cells lining the small intestine and leads to the disruption of nutrient absorption. One of the symptoms associated with coeliac disease is bloating, though there are other more severe symptoms. Increasingly bloating alone has been linked by many consumers with the consumption of wheat flour-based products, bread in particular, and this has given rise to condition described as 'gluten intolerance'. The formal diagnosis of this condition is not clearly defined and is often related to self-diagnosis by consumers (Mansueto et al. 2014). Often the condition is related by consumers to one type of bread and not another, or even a wheat type, which furthers clouds diagnosis of the medical problem, e.g. bread made with ancient wheat grains may be considered to be less of a problem. Unlike coeliac disease, gluten-intolerance is not seen as an allergic response and symptoms are more varied.

The manufacture of 'gluten-free' products has a long history, beginning with products based on wheat starch in which the offending protein had been reduced to a very low level through refining. Gradually as the interest and need for gluten-free products increased, bakers have developed a wide range of products for consumers using a diverse range of raw materials, mainly starches from those grains which do not contain the gluten forming proteins, e.g. rice, maize, and other starch rich plant sources (Capriles and Arêas 2014). The production of gluten-free products commonly requires special production facilities, not least to avoid the potential for cross-contamination during production with gluten-containing raw materials. At the very least segregated production areas and extensive cleaning regimes between production runs are required. Today it is more common to have a dedicated plant with appropriate measures to avoid the accidental introduction of inappropriate raw materials can be taken.

Some adverse ingredient and food responses may be linked with the absence of a necessary enzyme in the human digestive system for the metabolism of a particular compound. A well-known phenomenon which can be associated with the manufacture of bakery products is lactose intolerance. Lactose is a disaccharide found in milk and comprises a mixture of glucose and galactose. Sufficient quantities of the enzyme lactase are required to hydrolyse the lactose in the small intestine. Lactase deficiency is a common issue in some populations around the world and may also arise as the result of other intestinal illnesses. In the latter case once the intestinal illness subsides, so usually does the lactose intolerance.

Diabetes is perhaps now the most commonly recognised medical condition which requires the need for special dietary products. There are two diabetic conditions which require different control measures. Type-2 diabetes is the one which is most commonly recognised and linked with diet and the modification of bakery foods. The condition requires the individual to control the level of glucose sugar in their bloodstream. This can most commonly be achieved through careful management of the diet; in particular regulating the intake of 'free' sugars. Bakery products suitable for diabetics have been formulated by removing sucrose and glucose products and replacing them with other, more complex carbohydrates, such as those discussed in more detail in Chapter 6. As will be discussed below, the replacement of sucrose and glucose sugars with other materials is not simple, as most of the 'sugar replacers' do not have the functionality of the materials that they are replacing. In addition, there is the potential effect on the total energy levels of the alternative products and in particular, the risk that the overall energy contribution per 100 g of product may rise unless other compensatory changes are made to the recipe.

3.10 Anti-nutrients and Undesirable Compounds in Raw Materials

Many food compounds can have adverse effects when consumed to excess. Indeed, many of the vitamins and minerals discussed above, have potentially mild toxic effects if consumed to excess but the consequences are rarely fatal. The vast majority of the toxins encountered in food raw materials are entirely natural, some of which may have to be removed during raw material processing in order to make them suitable for human consumption. An example related to baking is sorghum, which is widely used as a food source throughout Africa (as porridge) but has the potential for use in non-wheat breads (Cauvain 2015). The hard, outer coats of some types of sorghum contain significant quantities of tannins (polymeric polyphenols) which give then a distinctive dark colour and discourage their consumption by birds. The tannins confer a bitter flavour to end products and reduce protein digestibility. They also have the potential for binding with iron and other elements, e.g. calcium, which limits the bioavailability of such elements in the human digestive system. To overcome the nutritional limitations of dark coloured sorghums, it is necessary to remove the coloured outer layers of the seeds, commonly by pearling (Dendy and Dobraszczyk 2001). Sorghum is also part of a group of products which contain cyanogenic glycosides, along with bitter almonds, lima bean varieties and cassava (manioc). Glycosides are based on a cyanide group linked indirectly to a sugar molecule. The release of cyanide from the raw material is facilitated through enzyme hydrolysis during processing and by boiling, especially with cassava tubers. Fermentation is also known to facilitate the release of cyanide from cassava (Montgomery 1969).

Undesirable elements and compounds may be accumulated by plants during their growing cycle. Heavy metals such as lead, mercury, and cadmium, have been of particular concern with wheat and other cereals, not least because of their potential implication with impaired brain functions. There are natural geographical variations in the concentrations of heavy metals in soils and these may be impacted by industrial emissions, or through the dispersion of waste materials as fertilisers. There is an increasing focus on such potential food contaminants, with positive action being taken to limit their accumulation as the result of agricultural practices. In wheat and other grains, the heavy metals are most associated with the husk or outer layers of the seed coat. Cleaning and pre-treatment of the grains before milling commonly leads to a significant reduction in the levels of heavy metals in products destined for human and animal consumption (Binder et al. 2018). The introduction of wheat 'de-branning' systems into modern mills has also made a positive contribution to reduce the levels of heavy metals finding their way into the final flour. Residues of pesticides and other agricultural chemicals, which may carry through to the final baked products, are strictly monitored and maximum permitted levels tightly controlled by local legislation; their potential impact on human health is complex and outside the scope of this book.

Cereal grains may be infected with a number of biological conditions which results in the potential development of mycotoxins, with the potential for them to find their way into the final flour. These natural 'contaminants' are primarily associated with the developing grains in the field, but the risks may be increased during storage prior to processing. Common descriptors of the typical contaminants in wheat are; ergot, a fungal infection producing black or dark purple sclerotia, *fusarium* head blight infections, bunt (*Tilletia* tritici) and blackpoint (associated with *Alternarai* spp. and *Cladosporium* spp.) (Williams et al. 2018). The development of mycotoxins in wheat and other grains is well-documented (de Koe and Juodeikiene 2012). Mycotoxins are secondary metabolites of a wide variety of filamentous fungi. Between 300 and 400 of the known mycotoxins have been identified as potentially harmful to human and animal health. Cereals and cereal products are regularly screened for mycotoxins and maximum limits set by local legislation (Alldrick 2018). Improved methods associated with raw materials harvesting, storage, and processing have reduced, but not eliminated the risks associated with contamination by mycotoxins. While the manufacture of most bakery products involves a heat-processing step, mycotoxins may be heat stable with the associated risks being carried through to the final product at the point of consumption. For example, the medieval condition known as 'St. Anthony's fire' was commonly related to the consumption of wheat flour which had been contaminated with ergot alkaloids through the milling process (Bailey 1928). The condition was initially associated with, 'a tingling and burning of the hands and feet, then a frightful heartburn', progressing through to convulsions and potential blindness. Even in relatively modern times, symptoms of accidental ergotism have been reported. It is worth noting that wheat and flour milled from it, is not the only potential source of mycotoxins in a baked product. Fungal infections and poor storage of raw materials post-harvest will lead to significant infections in many agricultural environments and with many field crops.

Raw materials produced using genetic modification (GM) have entered some parts of the food chain in recent years, though their application in foodstuffs has not been universally accepted and the topic of their potential use remains contentious in many parts of the world. Much of the debate regarding their use is based on the potential agronomic and environmental impacts, not least with regard to biodiversity. The limited studies to-date, have not suggested that the use of genetically modified organism (GMO) raw materials in the human food chain has introduced any potentially harmful or unwanted compounds. However, large sectors of consumers remain at best cautious, so that many bakery food manufacturers have opted to continue with non-GM raw materials, or where this is not possible to remove the raw material concerned from their recipes. For example, some individual UK bakers have opted for the exclusion of soya flour from their bread recipes, or specify that the materials must be certifiable and verifiable as non-GM.

3.11 Undesirable Compounds Which May Form During Processing and Baking

Undesirable compounds in human health terms, may form during the processing of raw materials to baked products; acrylamide is one such compound that has been identified and furan(s) another. It should be noted that both acrylamide and furan have always been formed in the cooking and baking of various foods. With the recognition of a potential negative impact on human health from such compounds, food manufacturers have sought to limit the level of their formation and in many parts of the world legislative limits have been set for their presence (e.g. The European Commission 2017). Given the natural nature of their formation, their complete elimination is unlikely, though mitigation strategies have been clearly identified and are being progressively implemented.

Acrylamide is a low molecular weight compound formed as a result of reactions that take place in starchy/high carbohydrate foods. The reactions occur alongside the Maillard browning reaction (Perez-Locas and Yaylayan 2010) and in the presence of asparagine, a reducing sugar (such as glucose) and heat (baking, frying, toasting, or roasting). Asparagine is a natural occurring amino acid present in some protein-rich raw materials of plant origin which includes grains and flours. It is suspected to be a carcinogen in animals and humans. The levels of acrylamide in baked products are very low and are associated with the crust formation in baked products. Its formation only occurs at temperatures above 120°C and so this means that any acrylamide which is present, is in the crust of baked products, since the body of bread and cakes do not achieve such high temperatures. Acrylamide levels can be limited by controlling the formation of its precursors by altering the mechanisms by which acrylamide is formed; e.g. by reducing the temperatures and time in baking, or reducing or replacing some of the acrylamide-promoting ingredients, such as the reducing sugars, in the formulation. It is claimed that when using some types of processing, such as prolonged fermentation, levels are lower. Acrylamide formation may be limited by the addition of ingredients such as free glycine (another naturally occurring amino acid), but it should be noted that adding high quantities of glycine to bread dough may lead to reduced yeast activity. It has also been claimed that the introduction of steam during the final stages of baking will help reduce acrylamide formation. This approach would have a significant negative impact on the crust formation of some types of crusty bread products, and is probably best suited to soft crust products. Enzyme preparations based on aspariginase from *Aspergillus niger* or *Aspergillus oryzae* bacteria, are available as part of an acrylamide reduction strategy (de Boer et al. 2005). These enzymes convert asparagines into another naturally occurring amino acid, called aspartate or aspartic acid, which means that the asparagine is no longer available for taking part in the acrylamide-forming reaction. It is claimed that these enzymes do not affect the crust browning or taste of the products, nor their nutritional qualities.

Furan (furans, methylfurans) are heterocyclic organic compounds which form during heat processes, such as roasting, baking, and cooking. They can form from a variety of food raw material precursor compounds, including vitamin C, carbohydrates, amino acids, unsaturated fatty acids, and carotenoids. In common with acrylamide formation, their presence in foods and beverages is unavoidable. Being relatively volatile compounds, the levels of furans remaining in foods and beverages varies according to the food preparation process. Knutsen et al. (2017) reported to the European Food Safety Authority (EFSA) Panel on Contaminants in the Food Chain (CONTAM) on the risks for public health related to the presence of furan and methylfurans in food, and concluded that there were health concerns associated with the incidental intake of furans. It was considered that the greatest exposure for adults was associated with roasted coffee and for infants, mainly with ready-meals based on margins of exposure (MOE). Furans were detected in bread, rolls, and other baked products, though the MOEs were lower than for coffee.

The acid hydrolysis of proteins during processing may lead to the formation of other unwanted compounds. One example is the compound 3-monochlorpropane 1,2-diol which is considered to be a potential carcinogen. Commonly referred to as 3-MCPD (and associated esters), it is most often associated with the preparation of Asian-style sauces, though the compounds may be present in plant-based refined oils, including palm oil. If present in processed oils which are used in the manufacture bakery products, then it is perfectly possible that 3-MCPD can be detected analytically in the final product. Commonly local regulatory bodies set maximum limits for the levels of contamination at or below those considered to offer no risk to human health. Detection of 3-MCPD is more likely in bakery products with high levels of processed oils in the recipe.

3.12 Conclusions

Wheat flour-based bakery products, especially those based on wholemeal flour (100% of the grain) have the potential to make natural and important contributions to the vitamin and mineral intake of consumers around the world. However, it is common for many types of bakery products to be based on white flours, which have lower concentrations of these key micronutrients. The widespread consumption of white flour based products, especially as various forms of bread, has been used as a vehicle by which to enhance nutrient intakes through the process of flour fortification. In some cases, fortification is aimed at the general population, while in other cases sub-sectors of the population may be targeted (as is the case with folic acid). Fortification is generally considered to be beneficial with no significant risks to consumers.

A range of ingredients which can make important contributions to the micronutrient intake may be used in the manufacture of bakery products and these will supplement the natural or fortified contributions. However, many of these raw materials are present in bakery products, other than bread and are less commonly consumed, so the overall micronutrient contribution to diets is modest, though still relevant. Such raw materials may be associated with the development of so-called functional foods, though their applicability in baked products may be limited by the very process of baking in the oven. In some cases (e.g. ancient grains), we are only just beginning to establish whether they have health benefits or not.

There are few negative health contributions associated with the basic raw material used in baked products (wheat flour). The significant exception is the presence of gluten-forming protein which promotes allergic reactions in some consumers. There is the potential for the primary and some secondary raw materials to deliver mycotoxins, a natural hazard, which requires careful management of the supply chain. In a limited number of cases, undesirable compounds may form during baking, but such compounds are now readily identified and strategies have been developed to manage them.

References

Adlercreutz, H. and Mazur, W. (1997). Phyto-estrogens and Western diseases. *Annals of Medicine* 29: 95–120.

Alldrick, A. (2018). Use of mycotoxin analyses. In: *The ICC Handbook of Cereals, Flour, Dough & Product Testing: Methods and Applications*, 2e (ed. S.P. Cauvain), 259–268. Lancaster, PA: DEStech Publications Inc.

Anon (2014). Homemade vitamin D. *Baking+Biscuit International* 06: 18.

Antonov, V.M., Staroverov, U., and Vorobjev, D. (2005). Bread made without flour Tonus – a high grade product for health nutrition. In: *Using Cereal Science and Technology for the Benefit of Consumers* (ed. S.P. Cauvain, S.S. Salmon and L.S. Young), 334–338. Cambridge, UK: Woodhead Publishing.

Bailey, A. (1928). *The Blessings of Bread*. London, UK: Paddington Press Limited.

Binder, E.M., Hubmayer, P., and Mitterer, G. (2018). Testing for animal feed production. In: *The ICC Hanbbook of Cereals, Flour, Dough and Product Testing: Methods and Applications*, 2e (ed. S.P. Cauvain), 305–344. Lancaster, PA: DEStech Publications,.

de Boer, L., Meermans, C.E.M., and Meima, R.B. (2005). Reduction of acrylamide formation in bakery products by application of *Aspergillius Niger* asparaginase. In: *Using Cereal Science and Technology for the Benefit of Consumers* (ed. S.P. Cauvain, S.E. Salmon and L.S. Young), 401–405. Cambridge, UK: Woodhead Publishing.

Burch, R. (2011). The stability and shelf life of vitamin-fortified foods. In: *Food and Beverage Stability and Shelf Life* (ed. D. Kilcast and P. Subramaniam), 741–754. Cambridge, UK: Woodhead Publishing.

Capriles, V.D. and Arêas, J.A.G. (2014). Novel approaches in gluten-free breadmaking: interface between food science, nutrition, and health. *Comprehensive Reviews in Food Science and Food Safety* 13: 871–890.

Cauvain, S.P. (2015). *Technology of Breadmaking*, 3e. Cham, Switzerland: Springer International Publishing AG.

Cauvain, S.P. (2018). *The ICC Handbook of Cereals, Flour, Dough and Product Testing; Methods and Applications*. Lancaster, PA: DEStech Publications.

Codina, G.G. and Bilan, E. (2006). Using inulin in bakery products. *Journal of Agroalimentary Processes and Technologies* XII (1): 225–230.

David, E. (1977). *English Bread and Yeast Cookery*. London, UK: Allen Lane.

Davidson, S. (1995). *Loaf, Crust and Crumb*. London, UK: Michael Joseph.

Davies, N.T. and Nightingale, R. (1975). The effect of phytate on intestinal absorption and secretion of zinc and wholebody retention of zinc, copper, iron and manganese in rats. *British Journal of Nutrition* 34: 243–247.

Dendy, A.V. and Dobraszczyk, B.J. (2001). *Cereals and Cereal Products*. Gaithersburg, MA: Aspern Publishers Inc.

Department of Health (1992). *Folic Acid and the Prevention of Neural-tube Defects*. London, UK: HSMO.

Dewettinck, K., Van Bockstaele, F., Kuhne, B. et al. (2008). Nutritional value of bread: Influence of processing, food interaction and consumer perception. *Journal of Cereal Science* 48: 243–257.

Dinu, M., Whittaker, A., Pagliai, G. et al. (2018). Ancient wheat species and human health: biochemical and clinical implications. *Journal of Nutritional Biochemistry* 52: 1–9.

EFSA NDA Panel (EFSA panel on Dietetic Products, Nutrition and Allergies) (2014). Scientific opinion on the safety of vitamin D enriched UV-treated bakers' yeast. *EFSA Journal* 12 (1): 3520, 19 pp. European Food Safety Authority, Parma, Italy.

Ehrnreich, H. (2000) Foods as medicine. *World of Food Ingredients*, June/July, 18–28.

Eve, L. (2000). Regulatory issues: Europe and Japan. In: *Essentials of Functional Foods* (ed. K. Schmidl and P. Labuza), 363–384. Gaithersburg, MA: Aspern Publishers.

Gil, A., Ortega, R.M., and Maldonado, J. (2011). Wholegrain cereals and bread: a duet for the Mediterranean diet for the prevention of chronic diseases. *Public Health Nutrition* 14: 2316–2322.

Hasler, C. (1998). Functional foods; their role in disease prevention and health promotion. *Food Technology* 52: 63–70.

Hegarty, V. (1992). *Nutrition: Food and the Environment*. St. Paul, MN: Eagan Press.

Knutsen, H.K., Alexander, J., Barregard, L. et al. (2017) EFSA CONTAM Panel (EFSA Panel on Contaminants in the Food Chain)). Scientific opinion on the risks for public health related to the presence of furan and methylfurans in food. *EFSA Journal* 15 (10): 5005, 142 pp. https://doi.org/10.2903/j.efsa.2017.5005.

de Koe, W.J. and Juodeikiene, G. (2012). Mycotoxin contamination of wheat, flour and bread. In: *Breadmaking: Improving Quality*, 2e (ed. S.P. Cauvain), 614–658. Cambridge, UK: Woodhead Publishing.

Korhonen, H. (2002). Technology options for new nutritional concepts. *International Journal of Dairy Technology* 55 (2): 79–88.

Mansueto, P., Seideta, A., D'Atcamo, A., and Carroccio, A. (2014). Non-celiac gluten sensitivity: literature review. *Journal of the American College of Nutrition* 33 (1): 39–54.

Montgomery, R.D. (1969). Cyanogens. In: *Toxic Constituents of Plant Foodstuffs* (ed. I.E. Liener), 143–157. New York, NY: Academic Press.

Owens, W.G. (2001). Wheat, corn and coarse grains milling. In: *Cereal Processing Technology* (ed. G. Owens), 27–52. Cambridge, UK: Woodhead Publishing.

Padma Ishwarya, S. and Prabhasankar, P. (2014). Prebiotics: application in bakery and pasta products. *Critical Reviews in Food Science and Nutrition* 54 (4): 511–522.

Perez-Locas, C. and Yaylayan, V.A. (2010). The Maillard reaction and food quality deterioration. In: *Chemical Deterioration and Physical Instability of Food and Beverages* (ed. L.H. Skibstead, J. Risbo and M.L. Andersen), 70–94. Cambridge, UK: Woodhead Publishing.

Rosell, C.M. (2012). Nutritionally enhanced wheat flours and bread. In: *Breadmaking; Improving Quality*, 2e (ed. S.P. Cauvain), 687–710. Cambridge, UK: Woodhead Publishing.

Schaarschmidt, S. and Fauhl-Hassek, C. (2018). The fate of mycotoxins during the processing of wheat for human consumption. *Comprehensive Reviews in Food Science and Food Safety* 17: 556–593.

Shapter, J. (1999). *Breads of the World*. New York, NY: Lorenz Books.

Siro, I., Kapolna, E., Kapolna, B., and Lugasi, A. (2008). Functional food. Product development, marketing and consumer acceptance – a review. *Appetite* 51: 456–467.

Slavin, J.L., Jacobs, D., and Marquart, L. (2001). Grain processing and nutrition. *Critical Reviews in Biotechnology* 21: 49–66.

Sofi, F., Whittaker, A., Cesari, F. et al. (2013). Characterization of Khorasan wheat (Kamut) and impact of a replacement diet on cardiovascular risk factors: cross-over dietary intervention study. *European Journal of Clinical Nutrition* 67: 190–195.

Taylor, J.R.N. and Awika, J.M. (2017). *Gluten-free Ancient Grains*. Duxford, UK: Woodhead Publishing.

The European Commission (2017). Commission Regulation (EU) 2017/2158 of 20 November 2017 establishing mitigation measures and benchmark levels for the reduction of the presence of acrylamide in food. *Official Journal of the European Union*, 21 pp. https://eur-lex.europa.eu/homepage.html.

Troncone, R. and Auricchio, S. (1991). Gluten-sensitivity enteropathy (celiac disease). *Food Reviews International* 7 (2): 205–231.

Wagner, A.F. and Folkers, K. (1964). *Vitamins and Coenzymes*. Oxford, UK: Wiley.

Williams, R.H., Bhandari, D.G., Hook, S.C.W., and Jellis, G. (2018). Testing cereals in the field and at the store and the relevance to end-product performance. In: *The ICC Handbook of Cereals, Flour, Dough & Product Testing: Methods and Applications*, 2e (ed. S.P. Cauvain), 47–78. Lancaster, PA: DEStech Publications.

Young, N.W.G. and O'Sullivan, G.R. (2011). The influence of ingredients on products stability and shelf life. In: *Food and Beverage Stability and Shelf Life* (ed. D. Kilcast and P. Subramaniam), 132–179. Cambridge, UK: Woodhead Publishing.

4

Drivers for Improved Health and Nutrition via Bakery Products

4.1 Introduction

The approaches used to convey nutritional guidelines to improve the health and diet of consumers vary in detail around the world, though the subjects of main focus tend to be common. Much focus has currently been directed towards issues related to global medical concerns related to the increase in the incidence of heart disease, raised blood pressure, type II diabetes and cancers associated with the human digestive tract and bowels. The medical evidence is clear that the underlying global increase in average consumer body mass represents a common factor in the increasing incidence of the medical conditions listed (Delpeuch et al. 2009). There are of course, many medical and lifestyle factors which contribute to the increased incidence of the named medical conditions and the rise in obesity. At the same time the overall life expectancy of individual consumers has been increasing and this is leading to an improved understanding of the role that food plays in delivering health and well-being as part of the lifestyle choices of modern populations. Understanding the contribution that food consumption makes to the health and well-being of consumers of all ages is fundamental to medical and nutrition experts alike, and is key to identifying dietary guidelines and targets which may be used in the development of new bakery products so that they can deliver positive health benefits to consumers.

Many consumers have varied diets during their lifetime; the nature of that diet may change in response to health and lifestyle changes and in many cases, to the development of specific medical conditions. The

Baking Technology and Nutrition: Towards a Healthier World, First Edition.
Stanley P. Cauvain and Rosie H. Clark.

consumption of bakery products commonly only forms part of the consumer 'normal' diet, with the proportion of the consumer diet which comes from baked products, varying globally and with the various consumer sub-sectors. In the light of medical concerns related to increases in obesity rates, many government-led nutritional strategies have focussed on the reduction of the contributions to the diet from salt, sugar and fat, and the universal desire to see an increase in the consumption of fibre by consumers. In this context attention has focussed on those bakery products which are high in recipe salt, fat and sugar, and low in fibre, with their potential negative impacts on health and well-being, and the role that bakery product manufacturers can play in delivering positive health benefits.

The nutritional guidelines as issued by the World Health Organization (WHO) (www.who.int/publications/guidelines/nutrition/en) provide a useful basis on which to discuss the place of bakery products in the drive for improved consumer health and nutrition. In the context of this work the relevant points may be summarised as follows:

- *Salt.* WHO member states have agreed to reduce the global population's intake of salt by a relative 30% by 2025, with the overall target being <5 g per day. Typically international averages have been quoted in the range 9–12 g per day, or around at least twice the recommended maximum level of daily intake. The actual levels of intake will vary widely according to consumer habits and government-led initiatives on dietary salt reduction.
- *Fat.* Food-based guidelines are related to not only the level of daily consumption of fat but also to the type of fats consumed. Broad guidelines for dietary fats intake are that they should provide around 20–35% of daily energy requirements. However, Elmadfa and Kornsteiner (2009) discussed the requirements for fats and fatty acids with respect to adults in a special edition of the *Annals of Nutrition and Metabolism* published by the WHO. The authors suggested that the minimum fat intake should be >15% of daily energy intake, while paying attention to an adequate intake of essential fatty acids.
- *Free sugars.* There is a conditional recommendation to reduce the intake of free sugars to less than 5% of total daily energy.
- *Dietary fibre.* The WHO recommends consumption of 400 g or 5 portions of fruit and vegetables per day to help ensure an adequate daily intake of dietary fibre. Subject to final international agreement on what constitutes dietary fibre, this then equates to around 18 g of non-starch polysaccharides per day.

- *Total energy.* The recommendations for total daily energy are inevitably influenced by geographical location, lifestyle, sex, and age, so that it is difficult to provide single values. In the UK the typical figure had been quoted for males as 10 500 kJ (2500 kcal) and for females 8400 kJ (2000 kcal), though these figures have been recently revised downwards by 20% for individuals seeking to lose weight. Similar values for total daily energy intake are recommended in many other parts of the world. Usually the daily energy intake values are related to age and activity of individuals. Most recommendations have the proviso that the daily energy intake level should be related to an individual's activity, with higher levels recommended for individuals engaged in significant physical activity than those with a sedentary lifestyle. Typically the difference between recommendations for active versus sedentary lifestyles is around 1680 kJ (400 kcal).

4.2 Dietary Contributions and Potential Health Impacts

4.2.1 Salt

Salt (sodium chloride) is not a nutrient and has no energy value, but does play a key role in human physiology and health. Its main function is related to the maintenance of the cellular membrane potential and it is associated with absorption of nutrients in the small intestine. Salt is commonly excreted in the urine, an effect which has been used to monitor sodium (salt) intakes in clinical studies (He and MacGregor 2007). While dietary salt does have a physiological role in humans, there have long been concerns regarding the level in the 'typical' human diet because of the widely reported links between high levels of sodium intake with hypertension, and other cardiovascular health problems (Elliot et al. 1996; He et al. 2014). There are number of potential sources of sodium in the human diet, though the main source is via salt, in part because of its profound impact on food flavour (McCaughey 2007) and therefore widespread use in processed foods, cooking and in the discretionary form at the dining table. Indeed, it is possibly the most powerful of the sensory impacts both in terms of 'saltiness' and in the enhancement of other food flavours. Salt plays a significant role in food preservation and safety, as well as a technological role in the manufacture of bread and other fermented products (Cauvain 2007).

In the drive to reduce the intake of dietary sodium there has been a strong focus on the role of salt present in manufactured foods in contrast with that of discretionary salt which is added by the consumer either during food preparation at home or with the meal serving. Estimates of the contribution to the diet of salt in manufactured foods and discretionary salt vary, not least because data for discretionary salt and home usage are not easy to obtain with any certainty. Salt levels in manufactured foods on the other hand can be measured analytically and associated with food purchasing/consumption data. It has been considered that as much as 75% of the daily intake of sodium originates from processed foods (Gibson et al. 2000) with around 35% being derived from bakery products (Angus 2007), though without clear data on discretionary use and intake data on food outside the home (e.g. restaurants and cafes) these data should perhaps be taken '*with a pinch of salt*'.

Bread is a commonly and globally eaten manufactured product which makes an important contribution to many consumer diets and thus has become a focus for moves to reduce dietary sodium intake. In the UK the establishment of the Consensus Action on Salt and Health (CASH) in 1996 set a basis for the reduction of salt levels in bread. With the collaboration of the UK baking industry, there have been progressive reductions in the salt levels in bread which has resulted in a significant overall reduction for bread and fermented products (about 50% of recipe salt), and to a lesser extent cakes, biscuits, and pastries. Similar strategies for salt reduction within the European Union have also been implemented, though a review by Kloss et al. (2015) revealed widespread differences in the levels of salt in consumers' diets. Other countries have taken the opportunity to legislate for salt reduction in bread and other foodstuffs (see for example, South Africa – Peters et al. 2017).

4.2.2 Fats

Fats and oils provide more than twice the energy per gram as carbohydrates and protein and are an essential and important part of all diets. They have many different roles in the human body, a key one of which is associated with the storage of energy. It is as a consequence of delivering this function that dietary fat has received particular attention over the years. The picture is complicated not only by the many types of fats and oils, but also in relation to their relevance in human nutrition.

A more correct way of describing fats and oils is by using the generic term 'lipids'. In everyday life we tend to think of fats as being solid or semi-solid and oils as liquid or fluid. These are simplistic descriptions since we can readily observe that solid fats become oils as the temperature rises and vice versa. Fats and oils come from a variety of marine, animal and plant sources and all have been used in the manufacture of baked products in the past. Today almost all of the sources of fats and oils for bakery product manufacture come from plants; there are a few exceptions, the most noticeable of which is butter. Despite the many consumer and health concerns regarding animal fats over the years, butter has retained its popularity in baked products, in part because of its flavour and sensory profile, and it part, because of its 'naturalness'.

For a detailed discussion of the chemistry and physics of lipids the reader is referred elsewhere (e.g. Stauffer 1996) but it will be useful to consider elements of fat technology which are relevant to the context of the subject of this book. The chemistry and physical form of lipids derive from the combination of glycerol combined with up to three 'fatty acids'. Most fats occur in the tri-(3) glyceride form, though di-(2) and mono-(1) glyceride forms are known. Most fatty acids have a linear or chain form and contain an even number of carbon atoms in their structure. If the links between the carbon atoms comprise single bonds, then the fatty acids chains are said to be 'saturated'. If, however, double bonds occur between carbon atoms, then the fatty acids are described as 'monounsaturated' for one double bond between carbon atoms and 'polyunsaturated' if there are two or more. To add to the complexity, the positioning of the carbon double bonds can lead to more than one fatty acid form; namely *cis* and *trans*. To further add to the complexity of understanding the nature and role of fats in diet and bakery food production, natural fats are a mixture of triglycerides, or put another way, a natural fat is a mixture of lipid fractions some of which will be solid and others liquid at a given temperature.

We can see from the above brief discussion on the nature of fats and oils why it is not possible to deliver simple dietary advice regarding their consumption and equally why the history of bakery product development with respect to fat type and level has been and remains, relatively complicated. The simplest dietary message has been and remains that the proportion of daily energy derived from fats and oils should be limited and this has in many ways led to the generic consideration of developing 'fat-reduced' bakery products; not least because of the positive link between fat in foods and fat, often excess, in the human body. Added to these general messages is the one that it is the level of saturated fats that should be reduced. Interest in the relationship between fat in the diet and cardiovascular conditions has attracted much attention over the years. For example, in the UK in 1984, the Department of Health and Social Security published a report on the diet of the nation in relation to heart and circulatory problems (Committee on Medical Aspects of Food Policy 1984). Known by the acronym COMA, the committee recommended that the total fat level in the UK diet be reduced to 75% of the 1984 intake (to achieve a preferred daily energy intake from fats of 35%), and that the ratio of polyunsaturated to saturated fats (p/s ratio) be increased to 0.45 (from 0.23). The publication of the COMA report was to lead to a wave of new product developments as the UK baking industry sought to deliver nutritionally enhanced product, at least as far as fats were concerned (Cauvain 1987; Barker and Cauvain 1994). However, not long after the publication of the COMA report the draft guidelines on nutrition labelling were revised to remove *trans* fatty acids from the saturated fat category.

As has already been noted, the manufacture of bakery and many other foods requires very specific technological functions from the recipe fats. In the fats and oils industry a process known as hydrogenation had been developed which allowed the modification of fatty acids to deliver specific functional properties. In principle there were two options, full and partial hydrogenation (Stauffer 1996). In recent years the concept of the chemical modification of fats has not sat comfortably with some consumer and retail sectors. These concerns were heightened with adverse medical findings associated with the consumption of *trans* fatty acids which were linked with increases in LDL (bad) cholesterol and reductions in HDL (good) cholesterol in the blood stream. Cholesterol plays a variety of roles in the body but as sufficient material can be synthesised daily by the liver, its ingestion is not a necessary part of the diet. The clinical implications of using *trans* fats in the diet were that they increase risks associated with heart disease, strokes, and type II diabetes (Stender and Dyerberg 2003). The industrial fat manufacturers' response to the concerns raised has been in most cases, to largely remove *trans* fats from their available products and to deliver the required technical functionality of fat products using alternative technologies, e.g. oil fractionation techniques. The industrial response has mainly been voluntary, though some countries (e.g. Denmark) have sought to use legislation.

4.2.3 Carbohydrates

Carbohydrates is an all-embracing term for food materials that are based on the presence of three types of atoms; carbon, hydrogen, and oxygen. As a generic group they are the main source of energy in most diets around the world. There are many raw materials and food ingredients which fall into the category of carbohydrates including simple sugars, starches, and fibres. The basic building blocks of carbohydrates are the monosaccharides, with the single molecules of simple sugars being linked in a variety of complex ways. It is these complex linkages which determine if and where in the human digestive system carbohydrates are broken down to provide the glucose molecules which are essential for the proper functioning of the brain, nerve cells and developing red blood cells.

Since sugars and fibre will be considered in separate sections below, attention will first be focussed on starch and its role in the human diet. The main sources of the polysaccharide that we call starch are the various plant materials that we consume. There are many rich sources of starch in nature, though in the context of the baking industry, the main sources are the cereal grains, especially wheat, which is processed into flour of various types. In the original grain the starch sits in the endosperm and provides a key store of energy which would be used by the seed when it starts to grow (Kent and Evers 1994). Starch is not a single molecule and is comprised of two forms; amylose – the long largely unbranched chain of glucose molecules and amylopectin – a branched form (Eliasson 2012). In the manufacture of many baked products, the exploitation of the swelling properties and subsequent gelatinisation of wheat starch is important in delivering specific characteristics in the baked product. Even after baking, the nature of the starch in some baked products is not constant and significant changes on product character may occur; for example, the firming (staling) of bread and cakes even in the absence of moisture loss is related in part, to changes in starch structure (Rayas-Duarte and Mulvaney 2012). Not all baked products contain gelatinised starch (e.g. biscuits and cookies) because the process of gelatinisation depends on a number of factors, including the level of water available and the potential influence of other recipe ingredients, most notably the levels and types of sugar. The importance of the effect of sugar on starch gelatinisation will be discussed below with respect to the potential for reducing sugar levels in baked products.

The significance of starch in the diet has perhaps, not attracted the same attention as some other macronutrients. However, that is not to say that the contributions of starch in the diet have been neglected. In the 1950s and 1960s starch-reduction in the diet was often prescribed as a means of encouraging weight loss, with an emphasis on limiting the intake of foods such as potatoes and bread. During that period there were a number of bakery product developments launched under the banner of 'starch reduction', though it was quickly realised that often such products contained more total energy per unit mass than the standard equivalent product. The Atkins diet which espouses a 'low carb' diet for weight loss is the most recent and perhaps best-known approach to reducing all dietary carbohydrates (e.g. Heimowitz 2014).

4.2.4 Sugars

Sugars arrive in the human diet from many sources, though by far the largest proportions are naturally associated with fruits. As with other carbohydrates, there are many forms of sugar, though the term is most commonly applied to sucrose, a disaccharide comprising one molecule of glucose and one of fructose. Sucrose is typically obtained from sugar cane or sugar beet and is available in a number of refined forms (Street 1991). Another well-known and used sugar comes in the form of high-fructose corn syrup and is obtained from maize (Pyler and Gorton 2008). The energy contribution of sugar is the same as that of starch and protein, $4\,\mathrm{kcal\,g^{-1}}$. All sugars are sweet tasting and have become a common part of many food products, not least sweetened bakery products, such as cakes, cookies, pastries, and buns. As noted earlier, the addition of sugars to bread varies around the world, though there are some fermented products like hamburger buns, where its addition is universal. When it comes to considering the role of sugars in the diet it has become common to consider them as either *intrinsic* or *free/added*. Intrinsic sugars are normally those which are an integral part of fruits and vegetables, while free sugars are those which are added by consumers and food manufacturers. While the latter classification clearly incudes sucrose, some naturally occurring sweeteners such as honey, syrups, and fruit juices also fall into this category.

The early nutritional and medical focus on sugar in the diet tended to be on the link with the incidence of dental caries (Mann 2004). Increasingly concerns began to focus on the contribution of sugars to the energy density of foods, with links with excess body mass and medical conditions such as chronic heart diseases and type II diabetes. The latter condition is perhaps the one most commonly associated with the negative health connotations of sugar. While much of the effect of sugar intake is considered to be related to obesity, it is becoming evident that this is not the exclusive negative health impact of high levels in the diet (Goran et al. 2015). Particular areas of concern have been related to sugary drinks and this is where much attention has been recently focussed. However, many bakery products like hamburger buns, cakes, biscuits and cookies, have not escaped attention and are increasingly, through their formulations, being identified as significant contributors to dietary sugars.

4.2.5 Fibre

As discussed above, interest in the role of fibre in the human diet has a long history with Burkitt (1986) reminding us that prominent physicians of many hundreds of years ago recognised the value of wheat fibre as part of a healthy diet. Kritchevsky (2001) comprehensively reviewed studies related to dietary fibre and the link with health issues such as obesity, diabetes, heart disease, and some cancers. Fibres are mostly polysaccharides which do not provide nutrient energy as they are not involved in energy metabolism at the molecular level. Their main role appears to be associated with gut health, with only a few types of fibre being broken down by the suite of enzymes in the human gut. In the context of bakery products, grain fibres (the celluloses and hemicelluloses) are the most common source, though other plant materials such as pectins (from fruits), gums, lignins (dried fruits), and pysllium (a herb-derived soluble fibre) find uses in bakery products. In some cases the fibre may be added for its technological function (e.g. pectin to stabilise gels) rather than its physiological function.

Definitions of dietary fibre which have been available to the baking industry have changed significantly in the last 50 years, moving from the concept of crude fibre to the more complex definitions of dietary fibre (Cauvain 2018). The complexity of defining dietary fibre has not made the task of product development easy for the baking industry. While obviously high levels of fibre are universally associated with wholemeal and similar breads, the position with respect to white or 'brown' breads is less clear. An example of the difficulties faced by bakers with respect to developing fibre-rich products revolves around the concept of resistant starch, the definition of which is covered in four different categories. Not all defined forms of resistant starch are present in all forms of bakery products, which hampers the understanding of what might or might not be determined analytically as dietary fibre, and how this may fit with any related nutritional data and what claims may, or may not be made. In broad terms the four types of resistant starch have been defined as follows:

- RS1 – considered to be physically inaccessible as part of intact or partly milled grains.
- RS2 – resistant starch granules in their 'natural' form as might be found in potato, green bananas, some legumes and high amylose starches.
- RS3 – retrograded starches from typical sources such as cooked and cooled potato, bread crusts and some flaked products.
- RS4 – includes a wide range of modified starches.

Some resistant starches occur naturally (RS1 and RS2), while others are formed during normal food processing (RS3), or by deliberate modification of the properties of a basic starch (RS4).

It is partly research studies and medical encouragement to increase the level of dietary fibre in the 'average' diet, which sustains the regular consumption of breakfast cereals and fibre-rich bakery products, like wholemeal and seeded breads. Despite the difficulties associated with defining dietary fibre in the last 20–30 years, the general recognition of the benefits of increasing fibre in human diets by health professionals has generated greater interest in the fibre-rich, flour-based products. When consumer interest in increasing dietary intake was combined with improved milling and baking technology, as was the case in the UK in the later 1980s, there was a gradual and meaningful increase in the quantity of wholemeal bread produced and being consumed. By the start of the twenty-first century, the proportion of 'non-white' breads (wholemeal, 50/50 white/wholemeal and seeded types) represented as much as 25% of all bread being produced. The interest spread to other fermented products such as rolls and sandwich thins (Figure 4.1) and for bakers launching new bread products, the development of 'non-white' variants has become an integral part of any new product range. The increasing interest in wholegrain products further accelerated the 'non-white' theme for new product development. Wholemeal bread had always been part of the bakers' product range, but it was only after the combined push of dietary advice and product development that the move to increasing fibre in the diet via bread products became a reality. With declining consumption of bread in some countries around the world, in part due to negative perception of the 'healthiness' of bread and its place in some diets, there is a risk that the previously positive messages related to fibre may be lost.

Fibre-enrichment in bakery products has not been universally implemented or accepted. There are biscuits and cookies where fibre levels are higher than with most other types, but generally the overall level of fibre in non-bread bakery products remains low. In part this is because the proportions of other recipe ingredients (e.g. sugar and fat) are higher than with many breads and this reduces the level impact of fibre-rich ingredients. Additionally, part of the lack of a wider range of fibre-rich bakery products comes from the fact that consumers may not equate products such as cake with 'healthiness' and higher fibre intakes. As will be discussed below, the introduction of fibre-rich raw materials may well deliver specific texture and taste profiles that consumers could find unacceptable for many types of bakery products.

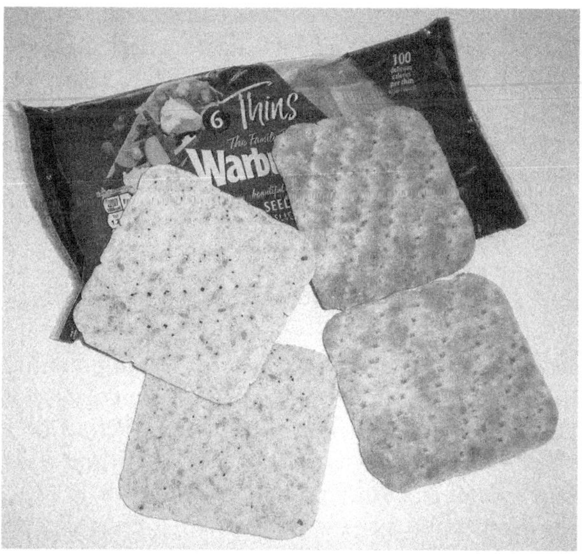

Figure 4.1 Examples of sandwich thins.

4.2.6 Satiety

While not a specific driver for the development of nutritionally enhanced bakery products, there has been much recent interest in satiety, the feeling of 'fullness' that comes following consumption of a meal. Fullness following a meal may of course simply result from consuming large (excessive) quantities of food but it may also associated with different food sources. Fibre and other lower energy dense materials are the ones most commonly associated with satiety. Recent evaluations of fibre-based slimming aids (Solah et al. 2016, 2017) have highlighted the role that satiety may play in managing weight loss. However, evaluating the satiation effect of different foods is not an easy task and requires the intervention of trained panels (Solah et al. 2015). As the study of satiety increases, it is reasonable to expect that the concept will play a greater role in the formulations of foods and contribute to the development of fibre-rich bakery products.

4.2.7 Glycaemic Index and Glycaemic Load

These terms describe the way food is digested by the body. The glycaemic index (GI) of a food measures its immediate effect on blood glucose levels over a short period of time following ingestion of a food. It is the blood glucose profile of 50 g of available carbohydrate in a test food compared to 50 g of glucose. The formal rating of glucose on the index is 100 and used as a basis for comparing the effect of all other foods. GI has been used as the basis for nutritionally enhanced bakery foods but has its limitations, not least of which is that it can only be accurately measured from a blood sample. It only measures the 'available' carbohydrate and ingredients that reduce digestibility, such as resistant starches, are not taken into account as they are digested later in the lower intestine. Fat and protein in composite foods can reduce the GI value, as can a lower pH and some aspects of food processing. The glycaemic load (GL) of a food is an expression of the potential impact the food will have on blood glucose levels. It is calculated by taking the percentage of the food's carbohydrate content per portion and multiplying it by its GI value, so that GL = (% carbohydrate per portion × GI)/100. GL measures both the quantity and quality of the dietary carbohydrates consumed. For example, the GL of one slice of a seeded loaf is only 8 while a slice of brown or white bread has a GL of 16. Cauvain (2017) gives GL and GL values for some typical bakery products. Low GI bakery products have mostly been associated with the addition of seeds and increases in the protein content of breads. Satiety has been linked with GI. Foods which are high in carbohydrates combined with a low GI take longer to digest and so give the feeling of 'fullness' for a longer period of time. An Index of Satiety has been drawn up (Holt 1998).

4.2.8 Protein

Proteins are commonly made up from around 20 different types of amino acids, though around 80 are known to occur naturally. The amino acids get their name because they contain at least one primary amino group (defined as $-NH_2$) and one carboxylic group (generally in the form COOH) which gives them both basic and acidic characteristics. While the human body can make many amino acids for the construction of muscles, there are a number which need to be taken in via food sources; these amino acids are often referred to as the 'essential' amino acids. Key sources of protein in nutrition are animal and plant products, but no single source of proteins can provide all of the essential amino acids required for human beings. Thus, a mixed balance of amino acids in the diet is important, whether it is animal and vegetable, or a mix of vegetable proteins alone. Proteins are used as a source of energy and they have the same energy value as carbohydrates, namely $4\,kcal\,g^{-1}$.

Given that many diets contain a mixture of proteins, there is perhaps less drive to nutritionally enhance bakery products with respect to protein content, though an improvement in the mix of proteins provided by bakery products may be desirable in diets where protein sources are limited. Commonly the approach for bakery products such as bread and biscuits, would be to add other sources of plant proteins to supplement the wheat flour. In this context soya flour is a popular choice (Liu 1977), in part because it is readily available and perhaps more importantly, it provides a well-balanced source of proteins considered to be of 'high quality'.

In recent years the interest in the protein and vitamin supplementation of food products has increased. Initially such supplementation was developed in the context of sports nutrition (Figure 4.2) but has more recently become part of the offering for mainstream bakery products. This has led to the formulation of some bakery products with the specific aim of meeting nutritional claims for 'source'

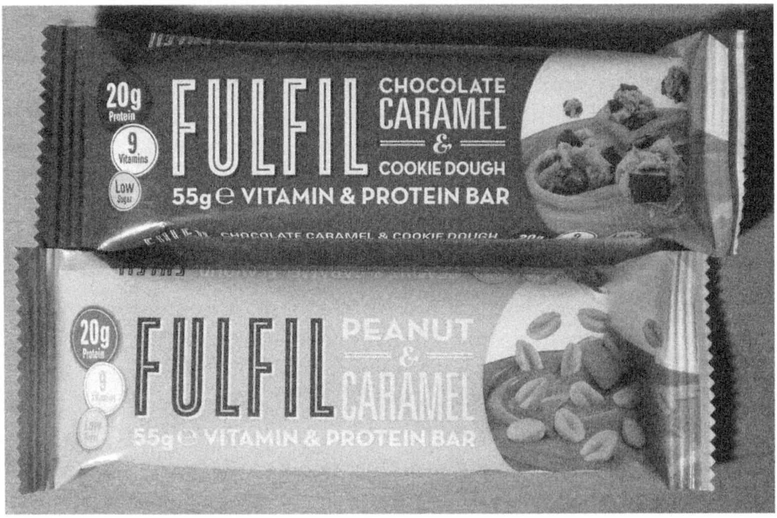

Figure 4.2 Example of sports nutrition bars.

(Figure 4.3) or 'rich source of protein'. In both cases it is likely that the products will need to meet specified dietary claims with respect to the daily contribution of the protein in the food and its contribution to total energy. For example, in the UK and EU to claim a source of protein a normal daily portion of the food must contribute 12 g protein and at least 12% of the energy content of the food.

4.2.9 Total Energy

When it comes to considering the topic of diet and health, the role of total energy intake is commonly the subject of nutritional guidelines in one form or another. Often the basic guidance comes from an institution or government department which has direct connection with those responsible for primary health-care in a given region; the UK example of a recommended daily intake values for energy and other macronutrients is shown in Table 4.1. The guidance data are commonly referenced according to the sex and to some extent, the age of individuals. Limiting total energy intake and balancing this with modern lifestyles which tend to be more sedentary in many parts of the world, has proved to be a difficult task and guideline values are subject to constant revision. In many advanced countries obtaining sufficient food is not a difficult task, provided that a suitable income is available

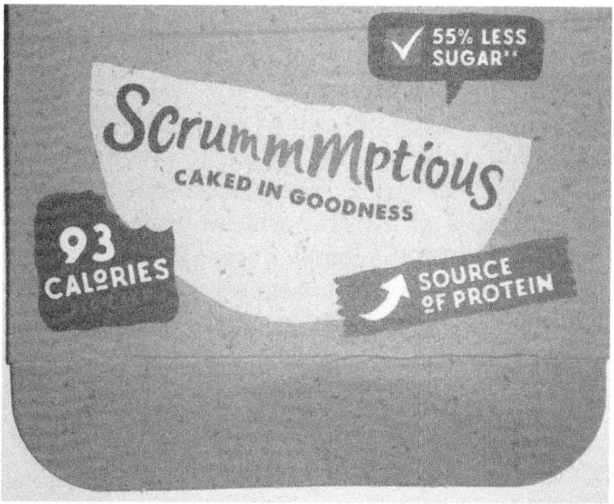

Figure 4.3 Protein-enriched cake.

to individuals, and this with changes in lifestyle (i.e. less manual labour), makes a significant contribution to the potential consumption of excess food energy in many parts of the world. In turn, this potentially contributes to problems of obesity and medical conditions which are exacerbated by excess body weight. Nutritional guidelines in many parts of the world commonly link energy intake with the need for regular exercise. While this may be a case of equating 'energy in' with 'energy out', there remains the need for delivering a suitable nutritional balance of macro- and micronutrients in the diet.

Table 4.1 UK recommended daily intake for energy and macronutrients.

Energy	2000 kcal/day (8400 kJ)
Total fat	Less than 70 g
Saturated fat	Less than 20 g
Carbohydrates	More than 260 g
Total sugars	Less than 90 g
Protein	50 g
Salt	Less than 6 g

Most of the macronutrients associated with raw materials make significant contributions to the total energy of a baked product. In the context of contributing to improvements to diet and health there are relatively few ingredients which can be used in significant quantities which make direct contribution to lowering the energy concentration. Water is the one macroingredient which carries no energy value but as has been noted above, the level of moisture which remains in baked products has to be balanced against the complex needs of product quality and shelf-life. Fibre in its various forms is one macroingredient which may be considered when looking to reduce the energy value of a bakery food, as can the low-energy fat and sugar replacers discussed below.

4.3 Lifestyle Choices and Bakery Products

4.3.1 Organic

The production of raw materials using organic methods of agriculture has increased significantly in recent years, though such materials still represent a relatively small part of total food production and consumption. The processes by which the raw materials are grown, processed, and manufactured into foods, are strictly controlled through established organisations like the Soil Association in the UK. In essence the structural integrity of the raw materials is the same as those for other agricultural methods; that is, the nutritional contribution of the macromaterials are not directly affected. Where differences may occur, they tend to be associated with residues of agricultural chemicals, which should be absent in the case of organic products. The formulation of organic bakery products will be essentially similar to that of non-organic, though there may be small differences in the ultimately contributions of the macronutritional ingredients. In some cases, low levels of specialist non-organic ingredients may be permitted, but these days many more organic alternatives are commonly available. The commonly held belief of some consumers that organic food is healthier was examined in a comprehensive review of the relevant literature by Smith-Spangler et al. (2012) and they concluded that as far as the underlying nutrition was concerned, evidence for health benefits was lacking, though they did recognise that the consumption of organic produce would reduce the exposure of the consumer to pesticide residues and antibiotic resistant bacteria.

4.3.2 Vegetarian and Vegan

Clearly those bakery pastry products which contain meat (commonly in pies) will not be suitable for vegetarians. However, vegetarian options for texturised, non-meat proteins do exist and can be readily used in the manufacture of vegetarian products (e.g. Quorn, see Figure 4.4), which may include bakery products. These days a large majority of bakery products have moved away from using animal fats (butter-based products apart) in bakery formulations in favour of vegetable oils based options and there is a tendency to base bakery formulations as much as possible, on vegetarian options so as to cater for as wide a customer base as possible. This usually means that no significant changes are required to many bakery formulations in order to meet vegetarian requirements.

Vegan requirements are more stringent than those for vegetarians and re-formulation to deliver suitable bakery products is more likely to be required. Many basic bread and fermented product formulations can be suitable for those consumers following a vegan diet, provided that milk and eggs are not included, along with the use vegetable oils and fats. This should not be major barrier to developing new products, given that egg and milk products have limited structural functions in

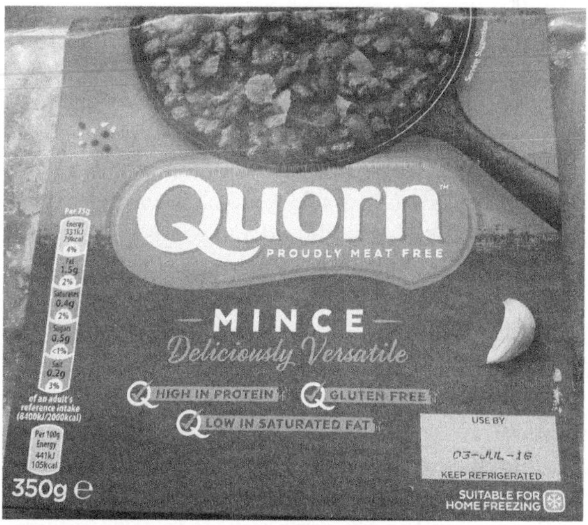

Figure 4.4 Example of a product based on Quorn.

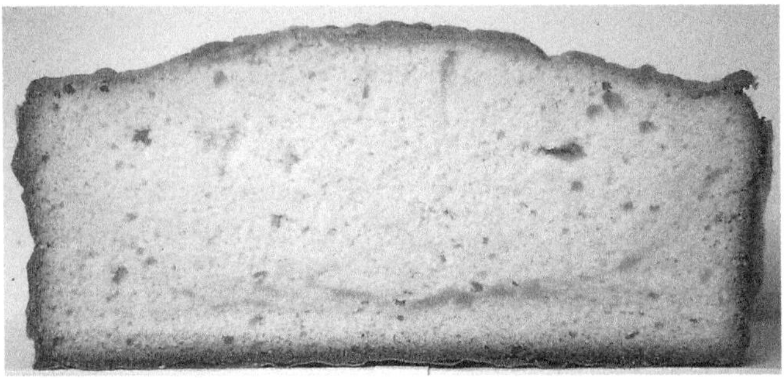

Figure 4.5 Impact of removing skimmed milk powder in cakes (note dark streak towards the bottom of the cake).

the manufacture of many fermented products. Replacing the flavour profile of egg, milk and butter (e.g. in brioche) is, however, a greater challenge and one which may not be easily overcome without some accompanying changes in product textural qualities. In some other bakery products, such cakes and cookies, the presence of egg and milk products does contribute to product structure formation and this means that significant product development will be required to meet vegan consumer quality expectations. In the case of cakes, the absence of egg protein can result in the loss of crumb cohesiveness unless that particular function is delivered with another source of protein. A number of replacement proteins have been suggested, including those derived from soya. Even the simple removal of dried milk products from cake recipes without relevant compensatory changes, can result in quality losses which consumers may find unacceptable. For example, the cake illustrated in Figure 4.5 exhibits a dark streak towards the bottom of the cake as a result of unbalanced liquid and solids levels in the recipe.

4.4 The Role of Legislation

Increasingly government-led health initiatives are providing drivers for changing the nutritional contribution of bakery products. In some cases the pressure has been based on a voluntary or collaborative approach. This was the case in the UK with respect to salt (sodium) levels in bread and other bakery products. It is worth noting that the

UK approach included the use of 'name-and-shame' tactics, with the publication of the results of government-led analytical surveys being used to show the relative progress of individual manufacturers and suppliers in meeting publically declared targets. This tactic, combined with retailer pressure, was particularly effective, since an individual company did not want the inevitable adverse publicity associated with not achieving the targets for progressive salt reduction. The role of the food retailers is further considered below. Similar approaches were used in the UK with respect to the removal of *trans* fats from bakery product formulations and are (as of 2018) being used with respect to sugar reduction in bakery products.

Other government-led approaches have been based on specific legislation to set nutritional targets and ensure manufacturer compliance. Examples of this approach include the action in South Africa with the setting of mandatory reduction levels for salt (see above). With the current significant focus on sugars in the diet, there has been much discussion related to the introduction of sugar taxes. Though much of the current focus has been on so-called sugary, soft drinks (www.beveragedaily.com/Article/2017/12/20/Sugar-taxes-The-global-picture-in-2017), the potential contribution for bakery products has not been ignored. For example, Public Health England included bakery products in its published strategy for reducing consumption and subsequent reporting of progress in 2018 towards its proposed 5% reduction target (www.gov.uk/government/publications/sugar-reduction-report-on-first-year-progress). While progress had been made, dietary sugar levels had not achieved the targets which had been set for 2018. The debate about whether such government-led indicatives will be successful in delivering specified dietary changes is outside the scope of this work. It is almost certain that dietary changes will not be achieved exclusively by single actions and that a more holistic approach will be necessary as noted by Gibson et al. (2017), with respect to the UK targets for sugar reduction.

Whether collaborative or legislative approaches are used to improve the nutritional value of bakery products is largely irrelevant, what is important to recognise is that re-formulations require manufacturers to consider the implications of changing not only their ingredient combinations, but also potentially their manufacturing processes (as is the case for example with salt reduction and the potential for increased dough stickiness). In addition to needing a proactive dialogue between legislators and manufacturers, there is a need to allow sufficient time to enable significant processing changes to be implemented. The financial implications for the manufacture of bakery products and possible impacts on consumers must also be taken into account if government-led dietary strategies are to be successful.

4.5 The Role of Food Retailers

In many parts of the world, food retailers are playing an increasing role in 'protecting' the healthiness of the consumer. Part of this trend is associated with the development of 'own-branded' or 'own label' products. Even though such products may be produced for a retailer by another manufacturer, the products will carry the retailer name and because of this, nutritional and product quality issues are commonly seen by consumers as a reflection of the values of the retailer. This places significant pressures on the retailer to ensure that their products have the appropriate image. Thus, in the UK, it was as much retailer as government pressure that added impetus to the salt reduction programme with bread. This was shown by the attitude to published government 'salt targets' in that once published, pressure was on the manufacturer/supplier by the retailer to meet those targets before the defined target date. Once again the pressure of the 'name-and-shame' approach could not be ignored. The desire of food retailers to deliver nutritionally enhanced products to consumers opens advantages for the development of new bakery products. It is not just a case of the baker having to respond to the various pressures around specific nutrition targets, but product manufacturers should be active in identifying opportunities for new product development because food retailers are regularly seeking new product options to offer consumers.

4.6 The Food Manufacturer

In the discussion above, one could have the impression that food manufacturers are not responsive to the development of their products with greater health benefits. Indeed on some occasions, in some quarters, the view has been that food manufacturers are not only resistant to change but are downright obstructive; such openly expressed views are at best misleading. Many food manufacturers will be considering and working on new products options on a regular basis, a number of which will certainly have associations with diet and health. Ultimately it is not in the food manufacturers' best interests to make products that consumers do not want to buy, or indeed which would do harm to their health. The vast majority of food manufacturers work within a prescribed legislative framework and are alert to consumer trends and interests and because of this, their need to improve or develop new products is as much a driver as any legislative or retailer pressure. A significant challenge for the bakery product manufacturer is the time that it may take to respond to deliver the development of a new product, the investment that may be required in setting up the relevant processing environment and all of the issues related to food safety and legislative conformance.

4.7 Conclusions

There are many drivers for improvements for the healthiness and nutritional contribution of bakery products to consumers' diets. Fortification with micronutrients is the driver most readily identified and perhaps the most easily achieved. Most commonly the driver will come from local or regional government-led interventions aimed at improving the overall health and well-being of the majority, if not all of the consumers in the region concerned. Government or institutional-led interventions may also be applied to the macronutrients in bakery products. This type of intervention is less readily achieved, as it requires clearly stated aims so that the sector of the food industry concerned is able to actively participate in the change and the introduction of nutritional changes to consumers. Because the manufacture of bakery products is based on the understanding of complex ingredient–recipe–process interactions, there is no simple route to follow. In addition to the dietary contribution of many ingredients which are used in baking, there is their functionality to consider, not just in the manufacturing process but also in the baked product after manufacture. Many opportunities may exist for the manufacture of nutritionally enhanced products but a key driver to their development is for bakers to be able to identify and meet those opportunities.

References

Angus, F. (2007). Dietary salt intake: sources and targets for reduction. In: *Reducing Salt in Foods: Practical Strategies* (ed. D. Kilcast and F. Angus), 3–17. Cambridge, UK: Woodhead Publishing.

Barker, P. and Cauvain, S.P. (1994) Fat and calorie-modified bakery products. *International Food Ingredients*, February/March, pp. 19–24.

Burkitt, D.P. (1986). Forward. In: *Dietary Fiber: Basic and Clinical Aspects* (ed. G.V. Vahouny and D. Kritchevsky), ix–xii. New York: Plenum Press.

Cauvain, S.P. (1987) Let them eat cake... especially if it's low fat. *Food Flavourings, Ingredients, Processessing and Packaging*, August, pp. 37–39.

Cauvain, S.P. (2007). Reducing salt in bread and other baked products. In: *Reducing Salt in Foods: Practical Strategies* (ed. D. Kilcast and F.Angus), 283–295. Cambridge, UK: Woodhead Publishing.

Cauvain, S.P. (2017). *Baking Problems Solved*, 2e. Duxford, UK: Woodhead Publishing.

Cauvain, S.P. (2018). Application of testing methods in flour mills. In: *The ICC Handbook of Cereals, Flour, Dough and Product Testing: Methods and Applications* (ed. S.P. Cauvain). Lancaster, PA: DES*tech* Publications.

Committee on Medical Aspects of Food Policy (1984). *Diet and Cardiovascular Disease: Report of the Panel on Diet in Relation to Cardiovascular Disease.* Department of Health and Social Security: Report of Health and Social Subjects No. 28. London, UK: HSMO.

Delpeuch, F., Maire, B., Monnier, E., and Holdsworth, M. (2009). *Globesity: A Planet Out of Control?* London, UK: Earthscan Ltd.

Eliasson, A.-C. (2012). Wheat starch structure and bread quality. In: *Breadmaking: Improving Quality* (ed. S.P. Cauvain), 123–148. Cambridge, UK: Woodhead Publishing.

Elliot, P., StamLer, J., Nichols, R. et al. (1996). Intersalt revisited: further analyses of 24 hour sodium excretion and blood pressure within and across populations. *British Medical Journal* 312 (7041): 1249–1253.

Elmadfa, I. and Kornsteiner, M. (2009). Fats and fatty acid requirements for adults. *Annals of Nutrition and Metabolism* 55: 56–75.

Gibson, J., Armstron, G., and McIlveen, H. (2000). A case for reducing salt in processed foods. *Nutrition and Food Science* 30 (4/5): 161–173.

Gibson, S., Ashwell, M., Arthur, J. et al. (2017). What can the food and drink industry do to help achieve the 5% free sugars goal? *Perspectives in Public Health* 137 (4): 237–247.

Goran, M.I., Tappy, L., and Le, K.-A. (2015). *Dietary Sugars and Health.* Boca Raton, FL: Taylor & Francis Group, LLC.

He, F.J. and MacGregor, G.A. (2007). Dietary salt, high blood pressure and other harmful effects on health. In: *Reducing Salt in Foods: Practical Strategies* (ed. D. Kilcast and F. Angus), 18–54. Cambridge, UK: Woodhead Publishing.

He, F.J., Pombo-Rodrigues, S., and MacGregor, G.A. (2014). Salt reduction in England from 2003 to 2011: its relationship to blood pressure, stroke and ischaemic heart disease mortality. *BMJ Open* 4: e004549. http://dx.doi.org/10.1136/bmjopen-2013-004549/ Available at: http://creativecommons.org/licenses/by-nc/3.0/.

Heimowitz, C. (2014). *The New Atkins Made Easy.* London, UK: Penguin Random House.

Holt, S. (1998) *Diabetes Interview,* May, pp. 1, 12–14. www.mendosa.com/satiety.htm/

Kent, N.L. and Evers, A.D. (1994). *Kent's Technology of Cereals,* 4e. Oxford, UK: Elsevier Science.

Kloss, L., Meyer, J.D., Graeve, L., and Vetter, W. (2015). Sodium intake and its reduction by food reformulation in the European Union – a review. *NFS Journal* 1: 9–19.

Kritchevsky, D. (2001). Dietary fibre in health and disease. In: *Advanced Dietary Fibre Technology* (ed. B.V. McCleary and L. Prosky), 149–161. Oxford, UK: Blackwell Science.

Liu, K. (1977). *Soyabeans: Chemistry, Technology and Utilization.* London, UK: Chapman and Hall.

Mann, J. (2004). Free sugars and human health: sufficient evidence for action? *The Lancet* 363: 1068–1070.

McCaughey, S. (2007). Dietary salt and flavour: mechanisms of taste perception and physiological controls. In: *Reducing Salt in Foods: Practical Strategies* (ed. D. Kilcast and F. Angus), 77–98. Cambridge, UK: Woodhead Publishing.

Peters, S.A.E., Dunford, E., Ware, L.J. et al. (2017). The sodium content of processed foods in South Africa during the introduction of mandatory sodium limits. *Nutrients* 9 (4): 404. http://doi.org/10.3390/nu9040404.

Pyler, E.J. and Gorton, L.A. (2008). *Baking: Science and Technology,* 4e. Kansas City, MN: Sosland Publishing Company.

Rayas-Duarte, P. and Mulvaney, S. (2012). Bread staling. In: *Breadmaking: Improving Quality,* 2e (ed. S.P. Cauvain), 580–596. Cambridge, UK: Woodhead Publishing.

Smith-Spangler, C., Brandeau, M.L., Hunter, G.E. et al. (2012). Are organic foods safer or healthier than conventional alternatives?: a systematic review. *Annals of Internal Medicine* 157 (5): 348–366.

Solah, V.A., Meng, X., Wood, S. et al. (2015). Effect of training on the reliability of satiety evaluation and use of trained panellists to determine the satiety effect of dietary fibre: a randomised controlled trial. *PLoS One* 10 (5): e0126202. https://doi.org/10.1371/journal.pone.0126202.

Solah, V.A., O'Mara-Wallace, B., Meng, X. et al. (2016). Consumption of the soluble dietary fibre complex PolyGlycopleX® reduces glycaemia and increases satiety of a standard meal postprandially. *Nutrients* 8: 268–280.

Solah, V.A., Kerr, D.A., Hunt, W.J. et al. (2017). Effect of fibre supplementation on body weight and composition, frequency of eating and dietary choice in overweight individuals. *Nutrients* 9: 149–163.

Stauffer, C.E. (1996). *Fats and Oils*. St Paul, MN:: Eagan Press.

Stender, S. and Dyerburg, J. (2003). *The Influence of Trans Fatty Acids on Health*, 4e. Publication No. 34. Copenhagen, Denmark: The Danish Nutrition Council.

Street, C.A. (1991). *Flour Confectionery Manufacture*. Glasgow, UK: Blackie.

5

Barriers to the Acceptance of Bakery Products with Improved Nutrition

5.1 The Nature of the Barriers

Before setting out to develop bakery products with improved nutrition or those which would be considered as 'healthier', it is as well to consider the potential barriers which may be raised for such developments. Considering the barriers at an early stage of product development should not be seen in a negative context, it is more the case that a consideration of the potential barriers at the start of the development phase is essential to understanding the route which needs to be followed to deliver a successful end-result. Much time and money can be spent on product development when the needs of the market have not been adequately identified, nor the opportunities fully explored. There are a significant number of potential barriers to the development of healthier bakery products and their nature will vary widely. McEwan and Sharp (2000) carried out qualitative research in the UK using both consumers and industry representatives, to consider the potential barriers to the development of reduced-fat bakery products. The results of the MAFF (Ministry of Agriculture, Fisheries and Food)-funded project, found that there were four key areas where barriers existed: consumer attitudes, product quality (technical), economic, and legislative issues.

A more detailed examination of the potential barriers suggest that they will be influenced to some degree by the bakery product sub-group of interest and the nature of the nutritional enhancement proposed; the more complex the enhancement, the greater the number of barriers which may be raised against the development. Accordingly,

Baking Technology and Nutrition: Towards a Healthier World, First Edition.
Stanley P. Cauvain and Rosie H. Clark.

we suggest and will discuss a more comprehensive list of barriers, they may be grouped under the following broad headings:

- *Government-led interventions*
  These are commonly associated with the fortification of ingredients in order to improve the nutritional value of commodities and products. While in most cases the need for fortification from a medical standpoint is readily identifiable and justifiable, it does not automatically follow that government-led interventions are totally accepted by all communities in which they are practised. In addition, there may be potential technical and practical barriers to the implementation of fortification in the manufacturing environment.
- *Legislative barriers*
  This area is often linked with nature of the claims which may be made with respect to nutritional and health benefits from specific ingredients, and the formulations of final products.
- *Consumer expectations and preferences*
  A wide variety of barriers will be raised by consumers and this is the most complex of all the areas to be considered for new developments. Consumer expectations from bakery products and therefore, the barriers related to nutritionally enhanced or healthier bakery products, will vary geographically and within regions, and between individual consumer groups.
- *Consumer and social barriers*
  While the consumption of bakery products is global, the influence of specific cultural or social requirements may make some relevant developments unattractive, or not possible.
- *Economic and commercial barriers*
  This is another complex area, in part dependent on consumer expectations. Some of the major issues that will need addressing by bakery product manufacturers will relate to the costs of adding specific 'healthy' ingredients, the costs of manufacturing changes and the financial positioning of the new product within the different markets.
- *Technological barriers*
  Technical barriers will inevitably be identified in the development of new products. Some may be overcome by available technologies, others by the application of new technologies while some may be insurmountable with available technology. Technological barriers can be many, varied and not inconsequential. They will be discussed in more detail in subsequent chapters.

- *Sustainability barriers*
  Many ideas for nutritional-enhancement of bakery products have their origins in scientific research which links specific nutritional benefits with a potential for use in bakery products. Often the healthy ingredients which are being proposed are not commonly associated with the large-scale manufacture of bakery products and existing raw material production may not be able to meet immediate demand or be sustainable in the longer-term.
- *Media-generated barriers*
  In a modern world were social and media communications are immediate, barriers can be quickly raised or indeed, broken. Increasingly this area represents a major challenge for manufacturing companies through ill-informed but widely read comments.

5.2 Government-Led Interventions on Fortification

As has been discussed in some detail above, the fortification of flour, and potentially other raw materials, intended for the manufacture of bakery products has a long history and is widely practised through government-led interventions for communities where the delivery of specific nutritional benefits have been clearly identified. Being government-led, this route follows a series of usually well-understood and practised interventions. While there have been and may continue to be, barriers raised against such practices, they tend to come from the medical and nutrition communities, rather than consumers in general. Barriers which may be raised may come from some consumer pressure groups as part of an informed debate and as such, should ensure that a well-balanced decision is reached before implementation of any food intervention strategy. Since such interventions tend to be associated with the fortification of basic raw materials (e.g. calcium in flour, iodine in salt) they are seldom seen as barriers in the context of new product development. However, mandatory fortification does not often present the manufacturer of bakery products with significant opportunities to make any specific nutrition of health claims and may account for the often 'lukewarm' reactions of commercial companies to such interventions.

Fortification of raw materials does not come without its practical barriers for the food manufacturer. The most readily identifiable example is that of flour fortification, which requires the miller to blend small quantities of micronutrients into flour streams running at high production throughput rates with a continuous flow of the base raw material which needs to be fortified. Over the years, flour millers have evolved increasingly efficient mechanical means of making the necessary additions to the continuous flour stream, though a challenge remains in ensuring that uniform blending of the micronutrients is achieved to the required analytical standards. In some parts of the world, fortification may be permitted or required in the bakery. In this case the required dosage in a batch-production system may be more readily controlled. In addition to the practical problems associated with fortification, there is always the issue of cost, not least in the context of who pays for the materials to be added. In a government-led intervention there could be a reasonable expectation that it would the government that carries the financial burden, however, this has not always been the case, and this may lead to barriers being raised by the commercial sector being mandated with delivering the required fortification. The on-costs of fortification may even be passed onto consumers through higher priced raw materials such as flour, or final products, such as biscuits. Fortunately, the levels of on-cost associated with fortification are relatively small when they are based on the quantities involved in the fortified material at the point of sale. Nevertheless, there is a cost associated with fortification and this may present a real barrier, especially with higher priced forms of nutrients and baked products with low sales prices. This may lead to some form of government financial support in delivering the required nutrition strategy.

5.3 Legislative Barriers

It is a globally common and fundamental requirement that any nutrition or health-related claims for bakery foods are significant and can be substantiated in defined scientific terms. Governments around the world employ various legislative means to regulate the use of ingredients and data in such contexts. The legislative requirements can represent a technical barrier to developing new, healthier bakery products, but one which is understandable. Clear definitions for what may or may not be claimed in health terms for bakery products, are widely welcomed by food manufacturers because they provide the guidance necessary for re-formulation of existing products and the creation of new ones. It is the 'grey' areas in legislation that create a significant challenge for food manufacturers. More often than not, these grey areas may arise not because the existing legislation is defective, but because legislation cannot anticipate outcomes from the medical and nutrition research in the future. In some cases, bakery product manufacturers may find themselves working towards new developments only for their activities to be overtaken by changes in government legislation or medical opinion. As discussed above, such a position was reached in the UK with respect to work being carried out on reformulation to reduce levels of fat in biscuit and cake recipes. This occurred when the classification of *trans* fatty acids as saturated fatty acids was changed (Ministry Agriculture, Fisheries and Food 1988; Food Advisory Committee 1988). In addition to the classification change there was a change in the nomenclature to be used, with saturated fatty acids to be described simply 'saturates'. While eminently sensible in scientific terms, such changes in descriptors were to have significant impacts on the presentation of information on the label of food packaging. Given that packaging must be prepared and ordered well in advance of food launches, the change could have had serious negative financial implications for bakery food manufacturers. Fortunately, the UK baking industry had been moving cautiously to developing reduced-fat products within the defined framework of that time and was readily able to implement the appropriate changes without significant financial disadvantage (other than the not unsubstantial costs associated with the product development programmes which were already in place and no longer viable). This particular example is an object lesson for the need of legislators and manufacturers to work together in order to achieve and implement sensible nutritional changes and in doing so, reduce the barriers which may be raised by manufacturing companies.

A potential problem which may be seen as a barrier, arises when a commonly accepted and widely used ingredient migrates from one food sector to another, especially when it is being used for the first time in the new food sector (e.g. bakery). This 'novel' use of the ingredient can result in the limitation of its use, at least until sufficient evidence has been assembled to support the case for its wider use in foods. In some cases, the barrier to the new application of an ingredient currently accepted for use in food may arise because of processing issues in food preparation. While consumption of a given ingredient may be acceptable when it is raw or boiled, the higher temperatures and often lower moisture conditions associated with oven baking, may cause the breakdown of the ingredient or its interaction with other recipe ingredients, leading to the potential formation of undesirable products related to human health and nutrition. Thus, it is advisable when considering the use of a less common raw materials in the manufacture of baked products, to seek out information and data concerning its behaviour during heat processing. This is not an easy task but one which may avoid the unnecessary waste of development time and resources. It is worth noting that the purpose of carrying out such surveys may not be entirely negative and indeed, may turn up some unexpected positive benefits.

An example of a hard barrier to the novel use of ingredients and raw materials is that implemented by the European Union (EU). As of 1 January 2018, a new regulation for novel foods, EU 2015/2283 (https://ec.europa.eu/food/safety/novel_food/legislation_en) became applicable throughout the EU. In previous directives on the subject, the EU was seeking to expand the categories of materials which would be considered as 'Novel' foods. The changes encompassed vitamins, minerals, food supplements and new food sources, such as insects. Also included were 'foods resulting from production processes and practices, and state of the art technologies', the latter including foods with 'intentionally modified or new molecular structure' which were 'not produced or used before 1997'. As well as attempting to react to the introduction of new technologies, the revisions were intended to improve 'conditions so that food businesses can easily bring new and innovative foods to the EU market, while maintaining a high level of food safety for European consumers'.

Not all legislative barriers are necessarily 'hard'. Some government approaches may be developed and applied on a cooperative basis with the manufacturers of bakery and other food products. Examples of this approach are the voluntary restriction on the levels of potassium bromate in breadmaking agreed between bakers in the USA in consultation with the United States Department of Agriculture (USDA) (American Bakers' Association/AIB International 2008) and the reduction in salt levels in bread by UK bakers in line with successive targets agreed with the UK Department of Health, discussed throughout this work.

5.4 Consumer Expectations and Preferences

Consumer expectations from bakery products vary geographically, and between consumer groups and individuals. Some of the expectations will be driven as the result of deliberate preferences, and some for historical, traditional, or ethnic reasons. The varied nature of consumer expectations for bakery products raises a variety of barriers in the context of nutritionally enhanced bakery products which are complex and hard to define. Where nutritional enhancement of bakery products (e.g. through fortification) has no discernible effect on the sensory attribute of the final product, there may be no significant consumer barrier. There is also unlikely to be a barrier where the nutritional enhancement has been practised for a long time and has become an integral part of the final product. Again, this is most commonly associated with fortification as would be the case, for example, with the continued calcium and iron enrichment of white flour in the UK, as legislated by the UK government since the 1940s. The major consumer barriers are those which relate to consumer expectations for the various categories of bakery products (as described in some detail in Chapter 2). It is often the case that the characteristics of 'healthier' bakery products are judged directly against the relevant standard bakery product; the problem is that the latter can vary significant on a global basis.

A comparison of bread recipes between developed and emerging economies illustrates this key point and shows that the move towards nutritionally adjusted bakery foods can only be achieved by adopting geographically local solutions. Examples of white wheat flour, pan bread formulations for the UK, mainland Europe, USA, Southern Africa, Australia, Indonesia, and the Philippines are given in Table 5.1. The formulations involved are relevant to the production of bread using no-time dough (NTD), sponge and dough (S&D) processes, the Chorleywood Bread Process (CBP) and Mechanical Dough Development (MDD).[1] These are the breadmaking processes which have been briefly described in Chapter 2 and the reader is referred elsewhere for the relevant technical details for each of these process

1 The term no-time breadmaking process refers to the practice of moving the bulk dough from the mixer to the divider without any rest period, in contrast to bulk or long fermentation systems in which the bulk dough is rested for a specified period of time after mixing and before dividing. Sponge and dough and other forms of pre-ferment systems are still essentially 'no-time' because after the second stage mixing of the sponge with the remaining ingredients, it is common for the bulk dough to move without a further rest period to the divider. A specialised form of no-time dough making involves the input of fixed energy levels during the CBP and MDD; essentially, they are the same process. The concept of no-time breadmaking processes almost certainly accounts for 50–60% of the world's production of bread.

Table 5.1 Some typical examples of white bread recipes throughout the world.

	UK	Europe	Australia	USA	Southern Africa	Indonesia	Philippines
Breadmaking process	CBP and NTD	NTD and CBP	MDD	S&D	CBP and NTD	NTD and S&D	NTD and S&D
Flour[a]	100	100	100	100	100	100	100
Water	60–62	58–60	58–60	54–58	58	58–60	56–58
Salt	1.2	1.8	1.8	2–2.3	1.8	2	2
Yeast[b]	2–4	1.8–2.2	2.0	2.4	2–2.5	1.5	1.5–2
Sugars	0	0	0	6	1.8–2.0	5	10–12
Fat	0–1	0–1	0–1	3	2.5	4	4–10
Soya flour	0–0.5	0	0–1	0	1	0	0
Milk solids	0	0	0	3	0.5–1.0	0–1	0–1
Improver[c]	0.5–1.0	0.5–1.0	0.5–1.0	0.5–1.0	1	0.5–1.0	0.5–1.0

[a] The recipes are simplified for the purposes of making total recipe comparisons. For example, the S&D processes split the flour into two separate lots for mixing (one for the sponge and the other for the dough).
[b] The form in which the yeast is used may vary from bulk liquid to compressed blocks to dried pellets. The essential difference is the proportion of yeast solids present (Cauvain 2015a). For the purposes of this table variations in solids/moisture content have not been adjusted.
[c] Improvers have proprietary formulations but typically contain low levels of ascorbic acid, emulsifiers, enzyme, and preservatives.
Source: Cauvain 2015a; Australian Export Grains Innovation Centre, personal communication; Cauvain, personal communication.

categories (Cauvain 2015a). The data in Table 5.1 are presented as bakers' percentage, taking flour as 100%. This approach to presenting recipes has been used by bakers for many years because many of the ingredients employed in bread recipes are added on the basis of 'improving' the breadmaking functionality of the flour. The bakers' percent allows an easy comparison of the anticipated breadmaking potential across a range of different recipes and processes. Some key differences emerge from the recipe comparison in Table 5.1. The three main ingredients of greatest nutritional significance in this work are salt, sugar and fat, and in Table 5.2 the data from Table 5.1 are converted to a nutritional profile of 100 g baked bread (assuming a standard 10% moisture loss during baking) to allow for more direct comparison of these key macro-nutrients.

A striking feature of the data in Tables 5.1 and 5.2 relates to the use of added sugars in bread recipes, ranging from no added sugar in the UK, mainland Europe and Australia, to modest additions in the USA and Southern Africa, and significant levels in Indonesia and the Philippines (in southern India recipe sugar levels are similar to those observed in south-east Asia). The technological value of adding sugars (commonly sucrose or high fructose corn syrup in the case of the USA) to bread dough recipes is relatively modest and it would appear that their 'historical' addition was established when having bread as a 'high-energy' food was more important than it is today in many parts of the world. While it is difficult to establish much of a positive functional case for adding sugars in breadmaking, there are negative functional effects arising from their addition so that reductions in added levels, ironically, can not only have nutritional benefits but may also bring about improvements in process and product attributes. However, today, product sweetness in many geographical areas is seen as a 'desirable' attribute and so reductions in added sugar levels present a significant hurdle to bread product redevelopment. Indeed, many consumers in parts of SE Asia describe bread without added sugar as 'sour' (Cauvain, personal communication), even when it has been manufactured with a process that does not employ a major period of fermentation, either in bulk or as a sponge.

Added fat levels also vary significantly in pan bread recipes globally as illustrated in Tables 5.1 and 5.2. Common positive benefits attributed to fat addition include aspects of improved crumb softness, eating quality and even flavour. Less well understood (though well-established scientifically; see Baker and Mize 1942) are the technological functions associated with additions of fat, especially when no-time breadmaking

Table 5.2 Comparison of salt, sugar, and fat levels in 100 g white bread based on example recipes given in Table 5.1 (for the purpose of calculation the mid-point of a range is used).

	UK	Europe	Australia	USA	Southern Africa	Indonesia	Philippines
Salt	0.80	1.22	1.22	1.40	1.18	1.29	1.21
Added sugars	0.00	0.00	0.00	1.24	1.25	3.22	6.64
Added fat	0.33	0.33	0.34	1.95	1.64	2.57	4.23

processes are used (Cauvain 2015a). Fat functionality in breadmaking is a complicated issue related to not only the level of fat addition, but also to the composition of the fat used (e.g. saturated, unsaturated) and in particular, the proportion of the added fat which remains solid in the dough when it reaches the oven. The data presented in Tables 5.1 and 5.2 make no reference to the compositional contribution of fat to bread, or any other baked product quality. The underlying chemistry of bakery fats is well documented (e.g. Pyler and Gorton 2008; Cauvain 2015a) and has been briefly discussed above.

The positive nutritional benefits of increasing fibre in the diet are well-known and have been introduced above. It is certainly the case that large particles of wheat bran, for many consumers reduces the sensory pleasure associated with eating bread. Alldrick (2001) drew attention to the complexities of developing dietary fibre enriched products and the need to balance the physiological benefits with consumer acceptance and purchasing power. Meuser (2001) too drew attention to the technological problems associated with increasing dietary fibre in baked products and illustrated examples of the sensory impacts of different types of bran and the treatment of wheat bran before it was used in dough making. In their reviews, both authors recognised the importance of product sensory qualities for consumer acceptance of fibre-enriched bakery products independent of the undoubted nutritional and health benefits.

While the consumption of higher fibre breads is an integral part of bakery product consumption in some parts of the world, it is not accepted universally by all consumers. For example, it is claimed that many children are averse to eating bread with 'bits in it' (a position personally observed with a child of one of the authors). This concept or barrier has resulted in the development of fibre-enriched breads using finer particle sizes and less coloured forms of fibres. For example, in the UK and elsewhere, there has been successful growth in products like 'half and half' and 'best of both' in which the dietary fibre is to some extent, 'hidden' from sight. In order to achieve such new products, developments in flour milling and baking technology were necessary in order to deliver sensory properties with fibre-rich breads more akin to that of white bread.

While the barrier to increased fibre consumption may be have been lowered in some consumer groups in some parts of the world, the same cannot yet be said for the majority of cakes, cookies and pastries. While there are significant technological barriers to be overcome related to the manufacture of healthier versions of these sub-groups of bakery products, there are greater consumer barriers related to the positioning of such products in the diet. For a long time, bread has been viewed as a basic or staple food consumed on a regular, often daily basis, though there is still the consumer expectation of sensory pleasure associated with eating bread products. The common basis for the consumption of cakes, cookies and pastries is somewhat different and more directly driven by sensory pleasure. In plain language, many consumers see the consumption of such products as an 'indulgence' or a 'treat' within their diet. In most parts of the world, cakes and pastries are not commonly consumed on the same daily scale as bread; often they are associated with other particular consumer practices, including being eaten with morning coffee, afternoon tea or as a desert after a meal. It could be argued that consumers have placed such products in a special space where indulgence overrides their dietary requirements. For such sub groups of bakery products, the barriers are significant and will only be overcome by meeting consumer sensory expectations combined with nutritional enhancement.

5.5 Consumer and Social Barriers

While nutritionally improved bakery products may be developed and become increasingly available, there is no guarantee that consumer acceptance will follow. Consumer preferences are often based on many of the product attributes discussed in Chapter 2. Expectations may be readily established through surveys, but the identification of the potential barriers for the purchase of nutritionally enhanced products remain complex and ill-understood. It may be that descriptors such as 'increased fibre', 'reduced salt', 'reduced fat', and 'reduced sugar' when applied to bakery products are themselves barriers to consumer acceptance, not least because they may subconsciously register as 'inferior' products with consumers, as least as far as taste and texture are concerned. The potential subconscious impact of a 'reduced' descriptor may be translated in a conscious impact on product acceptance by 'the violation of consumer expectations' (Szczesniak and Kahn 1971) as discussed below. A recent study by Kuhne et al. (2010), showed that European consumers placed great emphasis on the characteristics of traditional products, so that innovation activities designed to change the nutritional profile of such products carried with them the prerequisite that the traditional character of the products was retained. Where the ingredients delivering the traditional character make a major contribution to food structure, as is the case with the majority of bakery products, the innovation task will be greater and more complex.

The importance of texture in food acceptance was recognised by Szczesniak (1971) in a survey of 150 consumers to assess the importance of texture and flavour. Later work (Szczesniak 1990) was to emphasise that texture was especially important in foods with bland flavours; a conclusion which is especially important in the context of salt, sugar and fat reduced cereal foods, since reductions in those three ingredients are all significant contributors to food flavour. Measuring and understanding consumer perceptions and preferences for taste and texture is no easy task, not least because consumers cannot be considered to be a homogeneous group. Even in a given geographical area, there will be many potential variables related to socioeconomic background and historical influences, age, medical conditions and the processes associated with mastication (Smith 2004). Szczesniak and Kahn (1971) studied the awareness and attitude of adult consumers to food texture and identified many of the relevant factors. Amongst their conclusions they noted that texture could have both positive and negative impacts on consumer perceptions and that 'Texture awareness is increased when expectations are violated, associations are made with non-food items, or unpleasant mouth sensations are experienced'. Such findings emphasise the critical role that food texture plays in product acceptance and how important it will be for consumer acceptance when linked with the development of nutritionally enhanced bakery foods, where reductions in salt, sugar and fat result in texture changes in the final product. Potential negative changes associated with bakery food texture represent a significant and real barrier to the development of reduced salt, sugar and fat products, as has been noted above and will be further discussed below. For an introduction to the complex topic of consumer perception and preferences of food texture, readers are referred elsewhere (Meullenet 2004).

Both the historical and more recent social attitudes associated with the consumption of white rather than wholemeal bread, have been discussed above. It is somewhat ironic that the 'modern' trend of consumers in some parts of the world is to increase their level of dietary fibre through the increased consumption of wholemeal bread, or some other form of fibre-enriched bread. In some consumer communities the pendulum has swung to the extent that the consumption of white rather than fibre-enriched breads, is almost seen as 'socially unacceptable' and the latter are often (but not exclusively) associated with consumers placed in higher socioeconomic groups. Such changes represent a clear reversal of the historical position that the consumption of white bread was associated with an elevated status (and income) in society. Putting aside the status-related factors which are associated with non-white bread consumption, it is clear that some of the increased consumption of fibre-enriched breads is an indication that the 'health' message associated with fibre has resonated with large sectors of consumers, though sadly it may also be associated with the demonising of white bread (or any bread), often associated with the rise of the celebrity diet. Other social barriers which need to be taken into account when developing heathier bakery products include specific dietary requirements for vegetarians and vegans. They may also include the need to meet specific religious obligations in food production and consumption, whether on a regular basis or for specified calendar periods.

5.6 Economic and Commercial Barriers

This is another complex area and is in part, dependent on consumer expectations. Some of the major issues that will need addressing in the development of nutritionally enhanced bakery products will relate to the costs of adding specific 'healthy' ingredients and the subsequent financial positioning of the new product within the different markets. It is not unreasonable to assume that the introduction of nutrition and health benefits into bakery products will come at some cost. Even fortification of flour with basic micronutrients adds the cost of the necessary raw materials to the basic costs of the foodstuffs which will eventually be manufactured from the fortified material. It is not unreasonable to ask, 'Who pays such costs?' In the case of government-led fortification initiatives, the government may carry the costs or provide some form of subsidy for the manufacturer and consumer.

The position is somewhat different when it comes to the commercial manufacture of healthier bakery products in the context of the macronutrients. It is reasonable to conclude that the development of healthier bakery products comes with associated costs, many of which are not immediately apparent when project briefs are set at the beginning of a development. As has been noted above, the reduction in the level of one ingredient in a baker's formulation increases the level of all other ingredients in a given mass (e.g. 100 g of baked product). The total mass of ingredients passing through a bakery process is based on the number of individual bakery products required; the latter is referred to as the baker's 'yield' and relates to the unit sales potential of the product. Thus, there are costs associated with any reformulation to deliver healthier bakery products. They take several forms including:

- The inherent cost of the addition of a new ingredient in the formulation.
- The cost of a 'replacement' ingredient in contrast with that which it is replacing.
- The cost of the re-balanced recipe which may be greater (less commonly lower) than the standard formulation. This will include the possible consequences of using an ingredient to deliver specific health benefits which requires unintended adjustment of the product recipe to compensate for any negative functional effects of the new ingredient to deliver a consumer acceptable product.
- The cost of introducing new processing technology and equipment to make the healthier product.

Such cost-related factors raise the issue as to what price consumers are prepared to pay for enhanced nutrition or healthiness in bakery products. There will of course be some sectors of consumer populations that will be able to bear any extra costs involved, but there is also the assumption that large numbers of consumers will not be in a financial position or wish, to do so. In many 'political' environments, the current assumption tends to be that the baking industry should shoulder both the responsibility associated with the development and manufacture of healthier bakery products, and the associated costs of doing so. In some parts of the world there are arguments that 'taxes' on high sugar and high fat products should be used as a deterrent to their consumption (Williams 2016). Taxation may also be seen as a means of driving consumption of nutritionally 'undesirable' products downwards, but evidence for the efficacy of such an approach is equivocal (Evans 2018; Saunders 2018). Ultimately, it is the consumer who decides whether such approaches will work, though informed encouragement of government and other health-related agencies undoubtedly have a role to play (Sun 2017).

Consumer barriers may extend beyond the commercial cost barrier. One, often feared consequence of dual ranges of products (i.e. standard versus improved nutritionally) is that sales of the standard product will fall and not be replaced by sales of the new, healthier products, especially if the latter do not meet consumer sensory expectations or are higher priced. Such fears were partly behind the early reluctance of UK bakers to reduce salt levels in bread and it was only once industry concerted action was agreed that significant progress was made. In the early stages of the of UK salt reduction, a powerfully expressed view was that consumers' palettes would need to adapt to lower salt levels in bread and it was on this basis that gradual reductions over an extended period of time were implemented. It is certainly true that UK consumers began to adjust to less salt in bread, though a common comment was that 'bread began to lack flavour'. While this feedback may have provided some support for the increased production of more flavourful breads such as sour dough, the overall consumption of bread continued to decline throughout the period during which salt level reductions were being made. It is true to say that there has been a continuing decline in bread consumption in the UK and elsewhere (Anon 2014), over many years and there is no direct evidence that the salt reduction contributed to or increased this rate of decline.

It is more than likely that changes in process technology will be part of the technological package for delivering nutritionally-enhanced foods. A common experience with bakery product reformulation which involves adjusting levels of functional ingredients, is that the recipe becomes more sensitive in the manufacturing environment and this can lead to increased production losses unless modifications are made to production practices. Such issues can be solved but again, there will be an associated economic cost.

5.7 Technology Barriers

It has already been emphasised that product reformulation alone is not likely to deliver all the various nutritional changes being promoted by various agencies around the world and therefore, the successful development of the required bakery products will inevitably depend in part, on modifications to existing technologies or the development of new ones. The potential for increased process costs has been noted above; this most certainly would the case for major changes in processing technology and will represent a significant barrier in the product development process. In addition to the capital cost implications, significant investment in time will be required to first identify, then investigate the process options and finally move through the various prototyping stages before final implementation at production level. Ultimately it must be recognised that at a given moment in time, the technological barriers to delivering some forms of nutritionally-enhanced bakery products may be unsurmountable and may have to await the development of relevant processing technologies.

As noted above, a common implication of reformulating bakery product recipes is an increased sensitivity to processing variations. By way of example, we can consider the production of laminated products, such as puff pastry and croissants, and the potential to reduce the level of fat (especially the laminating fat) in the recipe. Some of these options have been discussed by Wickramarachchi et al. (2015) and include the need for improved control of dough processing temperature in order to maintain the layered structure required for the manufacture of reduced-fat puff pastry. There is also the potential for adjusting the number of theoretical fat layers created in the laminating process to complement a reduction in the level of the laminating fat. However, adjusting the number of theoretical fat layers during paste preparation is not without its limitations which in part, will be influenced by the nature of the processing equipment. Manipulation of the numbers of theoretical fat layers may be readily achieved with smaller-scale manual sheeting and folding arrangements than might be the case with some automatic plants. Thus, the intention to introduce a new processing option for the manufacture of a reduced-fat puff pastry item may well quickly reach the limits of existing technologies and require major changes to develop the appropriate new ones. As noted several times above, the key to delivering a specific bakery product quality is based on complex ingredient–recipe–process interactions.

In the case of laminated products, the sheeting process is especially important, and a critical interaction is that influenced by dough rheology. Cauvain et al. (2015b) drew attention to the importance of the contribution of flour quality in contributing to dough processing for both puff pastry and bread dough, including the important interaction between resting time for puff pastry between sheeting steps and flour quality.

5.8 Sustainability Barriers

Many ideas for nutritional-enhancement of bakery products have their origins in scientific research which links specific nutritional or health benefits with a potential for use in bakery products. Many of the 'healthy' ingredients which are proposed are not commonly associated with the large-scale manufacture of bakery products, and existing raw material production may not be able to meet immediate demand or be sustainable in the longer-term. Re-formulation to deliver healthier bakery products may invoke the 'law of unintended consequences', in that the agricultural sustainability of crops which deliver existing raw materials may be compromised when demand for them falls. While this is not a direct barrier to developing nutritionally-enhanced bakery products, it is still worth noting that in a global economy, changes in raw material demands do have consequences which extend beyond the immediate geographical area. Similar problems may arise when fat and sugar replacements are considered, in that the source of the availability of the proposed replacement may not be sustainable in the medium or longer-term without changes to agronomic or other manufacturing practices. The relatively recent moves by the food oils and fat industry away from fully- and partially-hydrogenated fats to palm oil fractions, and the potential loss of significant areas of tropical forest is a topical, though contentious example (Tan et al. 2009).

In many cases a proposed raw material for enhancing the nutrition of a bakery product is a by-product of some other manufacturing process. There are many examples in the scientific literature but all too often the proposers concentrate on the science and neglect the practical applications beyond the kitchen or laboratory scale. While by-products may represent an apparent good use of resources and deliver high quality nutritional benefits, in the medium- to longer-term the food industry must be able to obtain an adequate raw material supply to consider, let alone implement the addition of any such raw material.

5.9 Media Generated Barriers

While the media in its many forms, may not be seen as a direct barrier to the development of new and healthier bakery products, increasingly media attention represents a major challenge for manufacturing companies through often ill-informed but widely read comments. This particular challenge has become greater in a world where social and media communications are immediate and global. Such 'improvements' in communications means that barriers can be quickly raised and comment rapidly circulated. Today, we often read how images and negative comment on any topic can, in the modern vernacular, 'go viral'. In this context careful scrutiny of health-related claims needs to be undertaken during the product development process, along with any potential health risks which may be associated with the use of new ingredients to limit the potential for adverse publicity. It is therefore important that a thorough understanding of the relevant legislation regarding ingredient use is reached at an early stage of any new product development in order to understand and limit any potential negative media impact. The roles of the media related to the development of healthier bakery products are further discussed in Chapter 8.

5.10 Conclusions

There is a wide range of barriers to the development of nutritionally-enhanced bakery products, some more tangible than others. Legislative barriers linked with nutrition and food safety are perhaps the most readily defined as they are based predominately on data which can be easily verified analytically. Less well-defined but just as important, are the barriers which may be raised by consumers and social groups, not least because of the diversity of the former. Economic barriers may also form with respect to raw material cost inputs, the adaption of existing and the implementation of new process technology, and ultimately the price potential of the final product in the market place. There is no certainty that consumers will buy a healthier product at any price.

The recognition of potential barriers to a new product introduction in the early stages of development is an important step in avoiding unnecessary delays in the development process and in limiting the cost implications of projects which do not run to completion. Regular assessment of potential barriers throughout the development process is important as legislation and other relevant controls may change, as can health and nutrition-related information.

References

Alldrick, A.J. (2001). Developing fibre-rich foods in the twenty-first century. In: *Advanced Dietary Fibre Technology* (ed. B.V. McCleary and L. Prosky), 239–247. Oxford, UK: Blackwell Science.

American Bakers Association/AIB International (2008). *Commercial Baking Industry Guide for the Safe Use of Potassium Bromate.* Washington DC/Manhattan KS: ABA/AIB.

Anon (2014). Italy in the bread crisis. *Baking+Biscuit* 2: 62.

Baker, J.C. and Mize, M.D. (1942). The relation of fats to texture, crumb and volume of bread. *Cereal Chemistry* 8 (4): 672–676.

Cauvain, S.P. (2015a). *Technology of Breadmaking,* 3e. Cham, Switzerland: Springer International Publishing.

Cauvain, S.P., Cato, L., and Ma, J. (2015b). A review of some aspects of the practical importance of assessing flour quality. *Cereal Technology* 128–137.

Evans, C. (2018). How successful will the sugar level be in improving the diet and reducing inequalities in health? *Perspectives in Food Health* 138 (2): 85–86.

Food Advisory Committee (1988). *Nutrition Claims in Food Labelling Advertising.* London, UK: Ministry of Agriculture, Fisheries and Food/HMSO.

Kuhne, B., Vanhonacker, F., Gellynck, X., and Verbeke, W. (2010). Innovation in traditional food products in Europe: do sector innovation activities match consumers' acceptance? *Food Quality and Preference* 21: 629–638.

McEwan, J.E. and Sharp, T.M. (2000). Technical, economic and consumer barriers to the consumption of reduced fat bakery products. *Nutrition and Food Science* 30 (1): 16–18.

Meullenet, J.-F. (2004). Consumers and texture: understanding their perceptions and preferences. In: *Texture in Food. Volume 2: Solid Foods* (ed. D. Kilcast), 33–52. Cambridge, UK: Woodhead Publishing.

Meuser, F. (2001). Technological aspects of dietary fibre. In: *Advanced Dietary Fibre Technology* (ed. B.V. McCleary and L. Prosky), 248–269. Oxford, UK: Blackwell Science.

Ministry of Agriculture, Fisheries and Food (1988). *Guidelines on Nutrition Labelling. Drafted March 1985; revised January 1988,*. London, UK: HMSO.

Pyler, E.J. and Gorton, L.A. (2008). *Baking Science and Technology 4th Edn. Volume I: Fundamentals and Ingredients*. Kansas City, MO:: Sosland Publishing Co.

Saunders, J. (2018). Reducing sugar in our processed foods and beverages – will it make enough difference? *Perspectives in Public Health* 138 (2): 78.

Smith, A.C. (2004). Texture and mastication. In: *Texture in Food. Volume 2: Solid Foods* (ed. D. Kilcast), 53–81. Cambridge, UK: Woodhead Publishing.

Sun, H.-J. (2017). Efforts to reduce sugar intake: the case of Korea. *Perspectives in Public Health* 137 (3): 154–155.

Szczesniak, A.S. (1971). Consumer awareness of texture and other food attributes, II. *Journal of Texture Studies* 2 (2): 196–206.

Szczesniak, A.S. (1990). Texture: is it still an overlooked attribute? *Food Technology* 9: 86–95.

Szczesniak, A.S. and Kahn, E.L. (1971). Consumer awareness of and attitudes to food texture: I. Adults. *Journal of Texture Studies* 2 (3): 280–295.

Tan, K.T., Lee, K.T., Mohamed, A.R., and Bhatia, S. (2009). Palm oil: addressing issues and towards sustainable development. *Renewable and Sustainable Energy Reviews* 13 (2): 420–427.

Wickramarachchi, K.M., Sissons, M.J., and Cauvain, S.P. (2015). Puff pastry and trends in fat reduction: an update. *International Journal of Food Science and Technology* 50: 1065–1075.

Williams, S.N. (2016). 'Soda taxes' and 'fat taxes' can help tackle the twin problems of global obesity and under-nutrition. *Perspectives in Public Health* 136 (1): 21–22.

6

The Opportunities for Developing Improved Nutrition via Bakery Products

6.1 Introduction

The historical links between nutrition, health, and bakery products have been discussed above. As noted earlier, changes in the 'healthiness' of 'modern' diets is increasingly being questioned, with a popular notion being that 'processed foods' are a key negative contribution to health and well-being. All bakery products would fall into the concept of processed foods, with bread, cakes and pastries being early examples of both processed and convenient (as in 'ready-to-eat') foods. Bakers over the centuries have been aware of their contribution to the human diet but as might be expected, have responded to consumer demands for particular qualities in bakery products. Typically, fat has been used to deliver flavour, crumb softness, texture and pleasant mouthfeel, and sugar to deliver flavour (sweetness), crumb softness and shelf-life. The increasing focus on bakery products as negative contributors to diet and health may, at first sight, be regarded as a 'new product' opportunity, one waiting to be exploited by willing entrepreneurial bakers. Yet attempts to move in the direction of healthier mainstream bakery products have as yet, met with limited success. In part this lack of success is associated with consumer historical expectations of bakery product qualities and perhaps to a greater extent, the complex functional roles that the ingredients 'of interest' in health terms, play in the manufacture of bakery products. Some of those key attributes within the various sub-groups of bakery products have been identified above and it is through a better understanding of such qualities, combined with the

Baking Technology and Nutrition: Towards a Healthier World, First Edition.
Stanley P. Cauvain and Rosie H. Clark.

potential for processing changes, which will ultimately provide opportunities to deliver healthier bakery products.

In discussing the approaches for developing improved nutrition via bakery products, we must recognise that the opportunities will be constrained by local legislation, especially with respect to definitions, health claims and lists of permitted ingredients. This is a complex area well outside the remit of this work, but it will be necessary to include some relevant examples (and references) in order to develop key themes related to the potential development of healthier bakery products. Readers are advised to carefully check the relevant legislative constraints before undertaking the development of new products as there can be significant geographical variations in key areas of definitions and permissions. In some cases, formal legislation may be in place while in others there may be 'codes of practice' or industry-wide voluntary arrangements. An example of the latter is the progressive reduction in recipe salt in bread in the UK while in other cases (e.g. South Africa), mandatory reductions in recipe salt are in place. In addition to mandatory requirements, there may be special dietary issues with respect to the use of particular ingredients, some of these have been discussed in the relevant sections above.

6.2 Ingredient Declarations and Analytical Considerations

In most parts of the world, the manufacturer of bakery products is required to list the ingredients used in the preparation of the particular product. In the case of packaged goods, the information is recorded on the label, with the common practice being that the ingredients are listed in descending order of magnitude in the recipe before baking. While such information is particularly useful for consumers with respect to allergens, it does not provide the necessary nutritional information which consumers require in order to judge the relevance of that product to their diet and health. Accordingly, manufacturers include basic nutrition information to aid consumers in making their products choices.

A common (though not universal) approach is to include data relevant to:

- Total energy (calories)
- Total fat
- Saturated fat

- Mono-unsaturated fat
- Poly-unsaturated fat
- Carbohydrates
- Sugars
- Protein
- Dietary fibre
- Salt equivalent (based on sodium determination and adjusted accordingly to sodium chloride).

Typically, analytical values for the above components are quoted per 100 g, per typical serving, or both.

Ingredient listings and nutrition (analytical) data are commonly presented on the 'back-of-pack', see example in Figure 6.1. Such information may be supplemented by 'front-of-pack' information using simplified, more consumer related forms. In the UK and elsewhere, this may be colour-coded according to dietary recommendations. Often referred to as the 'traffic-light' system, it attempts to alert consumers as to the dietary position of particular products. In essence red indicates a dietary component which should be consumed sparingly, amber one that may be consumed more regularly and green one that may be consumed freely. The most common listings on front-of-pack information are for:

- Energy
- Fat
- Saturated fat
- Sugars
- Salt.

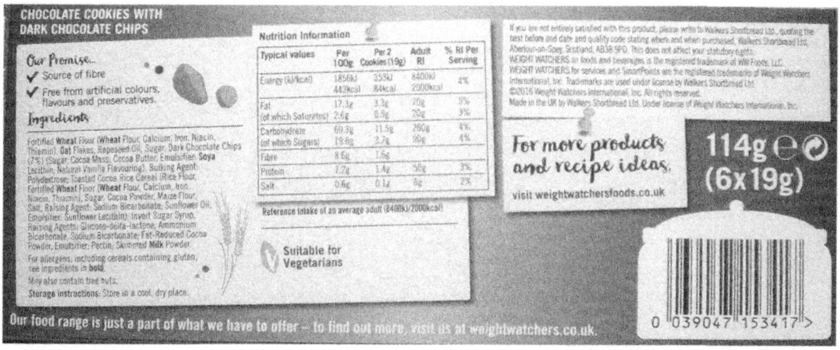

Figure 6.1 Example of an ingredient list and nutrition data for double chocolate chip cookies.

The format in which front-of-pack information is presented has not be universally adopted. A common format uses coloured flashes to specify the analytical quantity of a particular component per 100 g of product. The example illustrated in Figure 6.2 includes both analytical quantity and percentage of the Reference (daily) Intakes (see below). A similar approach may be taken with back-of-pack information (Figure 6.3).

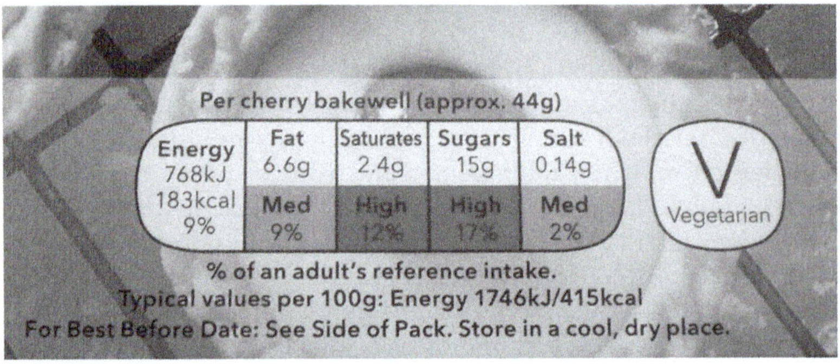

Figure 6.2 Example of front of pack nutrition data for Cherry Bakewells (comprising a shortcrust pastry, almond-flavoured filling and icing).

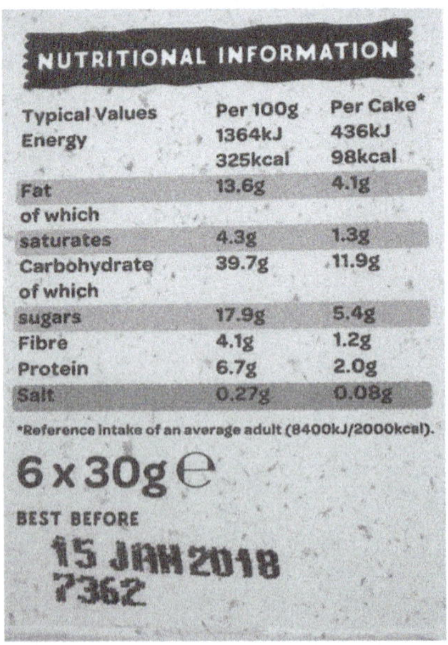

Figure 6.3 Example of back of pack nutritional information for cake.

6.3 The Reformulation Conundrum

For the baker the concern is less about the dietary profiles of particular ingredients and more about the dietary profile of the ultimate bakery products; though this is inevitably based on a mix of ingredients with their different nutritional profiles. When a bakery product has been formulated without immediate concern for its nutritional profile, then it is simply a case for the baker of meeting the local requirement for ingredient and nutritional labelling. However, when bakery products are to be constructed to meet specific nutritional profiles or match particular 'healthy' product images, the position is very different and in developing such products technologists have to meet head-on 'the reformulation conundrum'.

In many cases the reformulation of bakery products to meet individual nutrition targets such as less sugar, less fat, less salt or a specific energy target will mean that the proportion of the remaining ingredients will increase and while the individual ingredient target may be reached, a consequence of the reformation may be an increase in other 'unhealthy' ingredients, or total energy per unit serving or per unit weight. A simple example for a cake recipe will serve to illustrate the position. The basic cake recipe is given in Table 6.1 and the result of lowering fat, sugar, and both fat and sugar are illustrated in Table 6.2 using nutritional information. As the data in Table 6.2 show, a reduction in fat has a dramatic effect on reducing the energy per 100 g baked product, though the illustrated decrease does result in a small overall increase in product sugar levels. In contrast a reduction in recipe sugar has hardly changed the product energy levels, but has significantly raised the proportion of fat in the final product. Reducing both fat and sugar has inevitably delivered an enhanced nutritional cake (including higher protein) but critical to its acceptance by consumers would be the ultimate sensory properties of the product.

Because of their impact on the sensory qualities of baked products, with fat contributing to a shorter eating quality and sugar contributing to sweetness, there is a tendency to assume that nutritional reformulation is simply a case of using less of these particular ingredients in the manufacture of baked products. The simple nutritional reformulation of the cake recipe described above ignores the functionality, both in structural and sensory terms, delivered by the changes in ingredient levels listed in Table 6.2. Many bakery recipes are structured so that bakery technologists can appreciate the likely changes to product quality brought about by changes in the ingredient ratios,

Table 6.1 Basic cake recipe.

Ingredient	Ingredient weight based on flour weight (%)
Flour	100
Fat	57
Sugar	72
Whole egg	122
Baking powder	1.34

Table 6.2 Effect of compositional changes on the nutritional values for the basic cake recipe.

Nutritional properties per 100 g baked product[a]	Standard recipe	Fat reduced to 30 parts	Sugar reduced to 38 parts	Fat reduced to 30 and sugar 38 parts
Kcal	375	331	374	325
Fat	21.2	14.6	23.5	16.4
Sugar	18.2	19.7	10.9	11.8
Fibre	2.8	3.0	2.9	3.1
Protein	8.3	9.0	9.0	9.8

[a] Baking losses estimated as 8%.

with reference to the major building block of the product structure. In cake making the starch in the wheat flour delivers the major building block of quality and as such, the performance of the starch is directly affected by the concentration of sucrose in the recipe (i.e. the ratio of starch to water). In the example discussed above the standard sucrose concentration (derived as the weight of sucrose divided by the combined weight of sucrose plus water from all sources) is 0.41, while that for the reduced sugar recipe it is only 0.29; the quality impact on cake of such changes in sucrose concentration is illustrated in Figure 6.4. While fat is most commonly considered to contribute to mouthfeel (conferring a more tender eating quality), it also plays a functional role

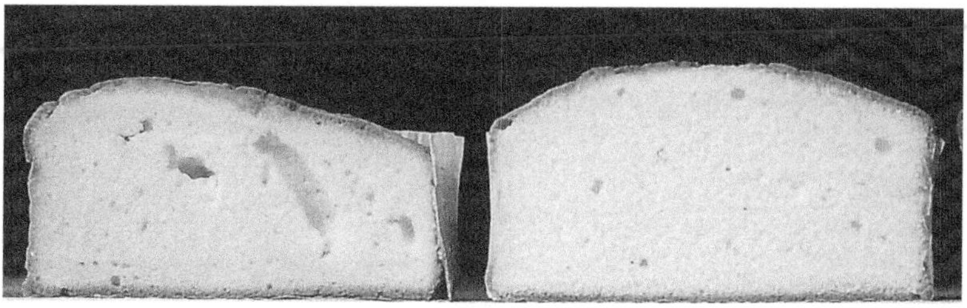

Figure 6.4 Cakes with sucrose concentration of 0.29 (left) and 0.41 (right).

and contributes to the mechanical aeration of many types of cakes, not least by affecting the balance between mechanical and chemical aeration and the delivery of an appealing product appearance. The impact of reducing recipe fat level is illustrated in Figure 6.5. Given that individual reductions in sugar and fat have negative impacts on cake product quality, it is inevitable that a combined reduction will deliver a cake quality of at least equally poor quality, without further recipe or process adjustment.

Cakes are not the only bakery products for which changes in recipe fat and sugar levels will have major impacts on final product quality. In the case of laminated products such as puff pastry, croissants, Danish pastry and crackers, the presence of discrete fat layers is a key determinant in the creation of a light and flaky texture. Further, it is not just the level of fat used in laminated products that is important, but also the physical characteristics of the fat employed. In a laminating fat it is the higher melting components which contribute most to the lift which characterises such products (BakeTran 2017). Unfortunately, the higher melting point components are also those which fall into the category of saturated fats, consumption of high levels of which are seen as nutritionally undesirable. In the case of cakes, it is also the higher melting point components which play the greatest functional role, in this case the 'solid' (higher melting point) fat making significant contributions to the aeration of the batter during mixing, with the fat crystals playing a significant role in trapping and stabilising air bubbles (BakeTran 2012a). In many types of cookies, sugar contributes to the flow, shape, and surface appearance of

(a)

(b)

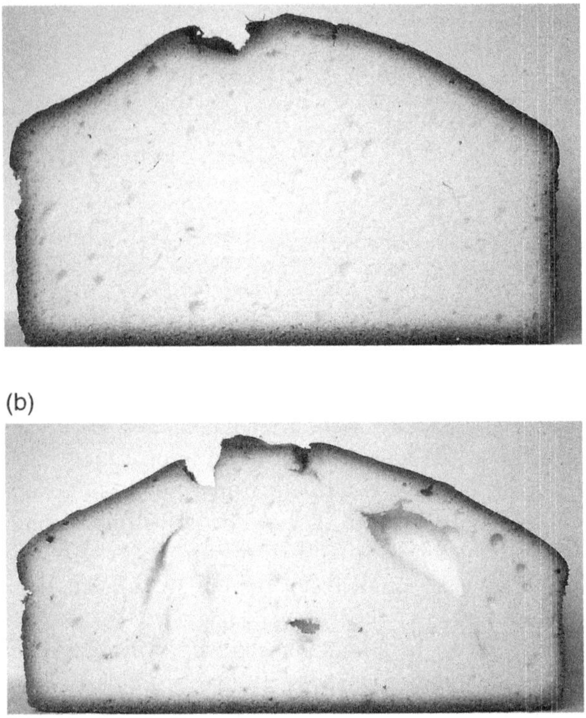

Figure 6.5 Cake with standard fat level (a) and 50% reduction (b).

the final products; for example, the surface cracking on many cookies depends on having the appropriate level and type of sugar in the recipe (Cauvain 2017).

6.4 Impacts on Product Microbial Shelf-Life

Another key consideration in the nutritional reformulation of bakery products is the potential impact on product microbial shelf-life. A number of categories of ingredients make contributions to prolonging the microbial shelf-life, including preservatives. In a nutritional context, two key ingredients are salt and sugar and when considering product reformulation, it is their impact on the product Equilibrium

Relative Humidity (ERH) (or water activity, a_w) that is of greatest concern. Weight for weight, salt is 11 times more effective than sugar at lowering product water activity (Cauvain and Young 2008), but in many bakery products the overall level of salt addition is significantly lower (but not unimportant) than that of sugar (sucrose). In considering ERH and shelf-life adjustment, it should be noted that while moisture and ERH are linked, they are not the same property when it comes to controlling microbial shelf-life. It is possible to have more or less moisture in a product without seeing major changes in product ERH (for a more detailed discussion of this subject see Cauvain and Young 2008).

The potential impact on the microbial shelf-life of reformulation to reduce fat and sugar is considered in Table 6.3 for the basic cake recipe given in Table 6.1. As expected, the reduction in recipe fat has almost no effect on product ERH, though the moisture content of the product has risen slightly. This is because fat has no direct impact on product ERH, but a reduction in its level has raised the proportion of water in the final product. On the other hand, the reduction in sugar has significantly raised the product ERH and as expected, has decreased the product microbial shelf-life. This is a relatively simple example of a major issue which must be considered when reformulating bakery products for enhanced nutrition and the compromise which may needed to meet nutritional targets. This simple example is not intended to show the necessary or available strategies for the extension of delivery of a particular shelf-life; readers are referred elsewhere for such discussions (see Cauvain and Young 2008). The prime purpose

Table 6.3 Impact of cake reformulation on its microbial shelf-life.

	Standard recipe	Fat reduced to 30 parts	Sugar reduced to 38 parts	Fat reduced to 30 and sugar 38 parts
ERH (%)	91.6	91.9	95.0	95
Estimated mould-free shelf-life (d)	4	4	<3	<3
Moisture content (%)	23.8	26.6	27.3	30.7

Baking losses estimated as 8%.

of this example is to illustrate how reformulation to deliver nutritionally enhanced bakery products may have unintended and serious consequences for other aspects of product quality. Mould-free shelf-life issues were highlighted in the example, but equally important are potential changes to sensory qualities with changes in ingredient proportions (further discussed below), staling (further discussed below) and texture (eating qualities).

6.5 Reducing Fat and Changing Type

In the pursuit of reduced energy bakery products, the recipe fat is most often a target for reduction or replacement in recipes because of its greater energy contribution compared with carbohydrates or protein. Diet and health concerns regarding fat may be associated with the sources, types of fat and methods employed in the manufacture of composite fats which may ultimately be used in the manufacture of baked products. A number of the key functional roles for fat in the manufacture of different sub-groups of bakery products have been discussed above and a knowledge of these form the base for potential approaches for fat reduction or replacement.

6.5.1 Recipe Fat Reduction

In some cases, fat reduction may be a simple case of identifying the lowest level of recipe fat that can be used without compromising final product quality. This approach in part, requires an understanding as to what the level of the most functional component must be to achieve the required effects. Usually the critical functional component of fat is its melting point or melting profile. For example, it is well known that the solid fat component is responsible for improved gas retention in bread dough (Cauvain 2015) and for air incorporation in cake batter (Cauvain 2017). In both types of product, the actual level of solid fat crystals required to achieve the required effects is small, but equally important is the uniform delivery of the fat crystals to relevant active sties in the dough (Brooker 1996) or batter. Thus, a common practice is to use an oil (liquid fat) to achieve the important dispersion function in the matrix during mixing. This dual functional requirement for fat may restrict the opportunities for an overall reduction in measured fat, but may offer opportunities to reduce specific types of fat, e.g. the saturated fats, which are also most often those with the higher melting points.

In terms of texture and mouthfeel, fat has a tenderising or softening effect. This effect has given rise to a common term for bakery fats, namely 'shortening', that is, its use delivers a 'shorter' texture to the final product. This particular quality applies to additions of oils and solid fats alike, though oils tend to lack the functionality of solid fats in the manufacture of bakery products. Thus, it is inevitable that reductions in recipe fat level will lead to textural changes for almost all bakery products, the exception being those forms of breads where traditionally recipe fats levels are low, and much of the texture depends on the degree and manner of gluten network formation.

Wickramarachchi et al. (2015) discussed the opportunities for reducing fat levels in puff pastry and laminated pastries in general. As noted earlier, in such products fat is used in a distinctive manner to convey specific textural characteristics and while the manufacture of products with lower fat levels is perfectly possible, the underlying textural characteristics are undoubtedly changed, often in a negative manner as far as consumers are concerned. Similar considerations apply to the manufacture of crackers, though fat levels tend to be lower than with puff pastry and so the opportunities for fat reduction in such products may also be limited. Similar considerations apply to many types of biscuits and cookies, in that fat reduction will lead to changes in product texture, with the products become harder. In this case the negative impacts may not be quite as severe as they could be with laminated products.

6.5.2 Changing Fat Type

The options for changing the type of fat are primarily based on introducing 'healthier' types of fat. As with many other bakery product reformulations, the balance is between introducing healthier options and retaining recipe functionality to deliver desired product characteristics. In the case of oils and fats there is no direct effect on the microbial shelf-life of the product, though changes in fat functionality may well affect product sensory properties and in many cases, the mobility and migration of water, especially in composite products (Cauvain and Young 2008). As far as energy contributions to products are concerned, both oils and fat contribute the same number of kJ (kcal) per gram of raw material. The background to the types of fat and their overall contribution to bakery products has been briefly discussed above, along with information related to types of oils and fats and their availability. In this section we consider some of the options for introducing healthier forms of fat into bakery product recipes.

Commonly the introduction of healthier fats into bakery recipes is based on changing from 'solid' fats to liquid fats (oils) at temperatures between 20 and 30°C. With such a generic change there is inevitably a loss of key functionalities; e.g. loss of gas retention in bread dough, loss of aerating power in cake batters, loss of lift in laminated products. The replacement of solid fat with oils often requires the addition of another ingredient to supplement the reduced functionality of an oil-based bakery product matrix; the most common introduction being the addition of a suitable emulsifier (see below). This is particularly true for cake batters and aerated creams, but can also be the case for bread and cookies.

With some products it may also be appropriate to introduce a process change which will improve the functionality of an alternative fat. To achieve this without significant change to final product characteristics requires a detailed understanding of bakery product processing. For example, by lowering the temperature at which laminated pastes are processed (sheeted and laminated) it is possible to use lower melting point fats (typically lower saturated fats) without compromising pastry lift at bake-off. This is achieved because the integrity and discreteness of laminating fat and dough layers is better maintained than would otherwise be the case at higher processing temperatures. However, lowering the processing temperatures comes with a need to make other changes, most notably a reduction in paste viscosity to compensate for an increase in the paste resistance to sheeting. Collectively, such changes in paste rheology require compensatory changes to be made to sheeting gaps, numbers of laminations and resting periods between sheeting stages (BakeTran 2017). Processing at lower temperatures is most commonly achieved using environmentally controlled conditions in the manufacturing area and if such controls are not available, costs will be incurred in their installation.

Similar process considerations may also apply where solid fat makes positive contributions to the occlusion of air during processing, and the retention and stability of the occluded air bubbles. In such cases it may be possible to move to less saturated fats by more closely matching the physical characteristics of the fat with the product preparation conditions. For example, in mixing cake batters the air occlusion stages in a multi-stage mixing method could be carried out at temperatures which optimise the functionality of lower melting point fats. Once again there is a delicate balance to be achieved since the fat concerned has to be plastic enough to be readily dispersed with the other ingredients and it must have a sufficiently crystalline nature to aid gas occlusion. This will almost certainly require the use of a composite oil/fat-based product to deliver the required blend of characteristics, even when the processing temperature has been adjusted.

6.5.3 Fat Replacement

Many ingredients are described as 'fat-replacers' in technical literature, they include:

- Lipase enzymes
- Emulsifiers
- Carbohydrate-based replacers
- Protein-based replacers
- Fat/lipid-based replacers.

Too often fat replacement has been seen as a matter of using a material with fewer kJ (kcal) per gram of material and simply 'mimicking' mouth-feel by using a material to 'bind' or increase product moisture content to deliver a softer mouthfeel (e.g. gums). In the case of energy reduction, the impact of many fat replacers is not as great as might be imagined and in many cases, the overall reduction in product energy density is relatively modest. However, in a complex recipe reformulation exercise, a relatively modest energy density reduction by such means may still make an important contribution to the product development project. A particularly useful contribution to product energy reduction comes from increasing recipe water levels, something often associated with the concept of fat replacement as noted above. However, a major problem associated with increases in product moisture content is the potentially negative effect on product microbial shelf-life which necessitates the introduction of other compensatory ingredients, process changes or alternative packaging technologies, such as gas flushing or control of moisture vapour transpiration rates (Cauvain 2017).

A common problem with fat replacers is that they are offered on the basis of changing mouthfeel in liquid or semi-solid food products. In contrast, bakery products (with the exception of many of their cream fillings or toppings) are solid foods and as discussed above, recipe fats make an essential contribution to product structure and texture beyond that of simply conferring a softer mouthfeel. This often limits the potential role for fat replacers in the delivery of reduced-fat bakery products. The potential types of fat replacers are discussed below. A common approach to their use in bakery products would be based on combining their effects with other materials in order to deliver an overall reduction in recipe fat in bakery products, while limiting any potential negative impact on eating qualities.

6.5.4 Lipase Enzymes

Fat replacement with lipase enzymes is most often seen in bread products where the recipe fat level is very low. The concept is based on particular lipase enzymes breaking down lipids (oil and fats) in the recipe (added or present in the ingredients used). The action is one of progressively breaking down the triglycerides to diglycerides and finally, to monoglycerides (Kornbrust et al. 2012), with the di- and monoglycerides conferring some of the required functional effects (e.g. gas retention in the dough), as well as the potential for reducing staling (see below). In many parts of the world, the additions of enzymes are considered to be 'processing aids' and as such, they are not required to be declared on the ingredient listing. This premise is based on the concept that these particular ingredients are denatured during baking and thus do not survive in their original form in the final product. Such considerations have given rise to the marketing concept of 'clean labelling' with respect to bread improver composition, however, it should be noted that this concept has no legal standing.

6.5.5 Emulsifiers

It is well-known with respect to bread products, that the addition of some emulsifiers will confer a similar functionality to fat in breadmaking, that is, they improve dough gas retention, subsequently product volume crumb softness and aspects of product cell structure (Cauvain 2015). In this case different emulsifiers deliver differing degrees of functionality. In bread the most commonly used emulsifiers for improving dough gas retention are the data-esters (Datem, di-acetyltartaric ester of monoglycerides), or sodium steroyl-2-lactate (SSL) (Whitehurst 2004), with the latter becoming less popular in some parts of the world as the result of increased focus on reducing the sodium (salt) level in baked products. While some emulsifiers will deliver improvements in dough gas retention and therefore bread volume, the mechanisms by which they achieve such improvements are not the same as that for fat. Unlike compound bakery fats, emulsifiers make the transition from solid to liquid quite quickly, usually at temperatures only achieved when the dough has been in the oven for some while. This is consistent with the need in breadmaking for a 'solid' fat component in the dough at the end of proof, but it may mean that some control of gas bubble coalescence that compound fats exert because of their 'gradual' melting profile, is lost as the dough temperature passes from 40 to over 60°C. The nutritional opportunities offered by replacing a bakery fat with an emulsifier are limited in bread because of the relatively low levels of fat. As noted earlier, the level of recipe fat does vary significantly and so in some parts of the world, the opportunity to use an emulsifier in a 'fat sparing role' does vary. Even so the fat sparing role for emulsifiers in fermented products will only make modest positive contributions to product healthiness, such as small reductions in product energy density and in some cases, saturated fat levels.

The potential for using emulsifiers in a fat sparing role is greater in the case of cakes as typically, recipe fat levels are a larger proportion of the overall product. Commonly emulsifiers are used in cake making where foam promotion and stabilisation are essential in delivering the required textural characteristics. Commonly, the emulsifiers used are the mono- and di-glycerides, polyglycerol esters propylene glycol fatty acid esters. Partial replacement of fat with emulsifiers in the manufacture of biscuits and cookies changes the paste rheology and the loss of the softening effect of the fat often requires an increase in the recipe water level to facilitate normal processing. This will in turn, require adjustments to be made to the baking process in order ensure that a low final product moisture content is achieved, and checking is avoided. Even where fat reduction in biscuits and cookies is achieved there will be some changes in product texture; often the final texture is harder and less short-eating, as shown in the example data in Figure 6.6. The potential for using emulsifiers to replace part of the fat in laminated products has been discussed by Wickramarachchi et al. (2015). The position is slightly different from that with biscuits and

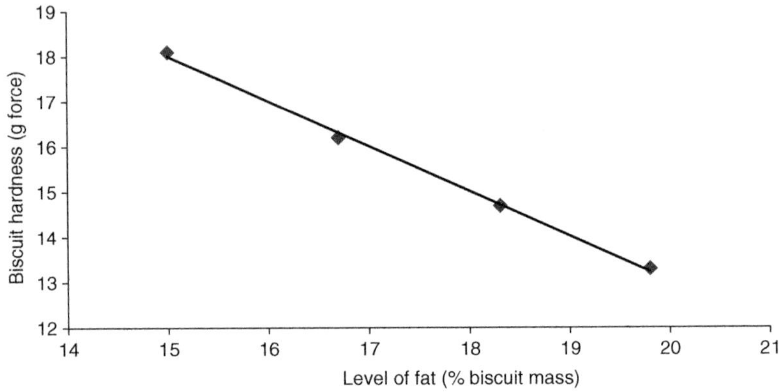

Figure 6.6 Impact of fat reduction on the hardness of short dough biscuits.

cookies, in that most of the recipe fat is not mixed throughout the paste but introduced through the typical sheeting and laminating effects as described above. However, fat sparing with emulsifiers can still bring about changes in texture as illustrated by the data in Figure 6.7. With the addition of DATA and SSL emulsifiers the firmness of the baked pastry decreases (i.e. the pastry becomes more soft to eat), with only part of the effect being attributable to increases in pastry specific height. The implication of such effects is that pastry height could be maintained by replacing part of the recipe fat with smaller quantity of an emulsifier.

6.5.6 Carbohydrate-Based Replacers

The most common forms of carbohydrate-based fat replacers are fibres. Their effect is based on the ability of fibre to hold water, thus mimicking the mouth-feel effect of fat in the final product. However, as noted above, the introduction of extra recipe water is not without its problems, not least with respect to product microbial shelf-life. In most cases, the energy contribution of carbohydrate-based replacers is significantly less than that of the fat that they are replacing, though the overall impact on the energy density of the final product depends on the level of fat being replaced and the level of addition of the replacer. Often it is the reduction in recipe fat that makes the most significant contribution to product energy reduction.

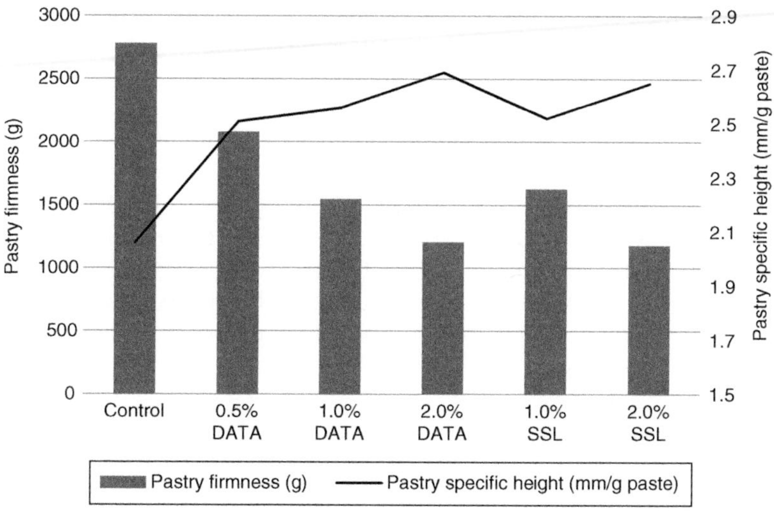

Figure 6.7 Effects of DATA and SSL emulsifier addition in the manufacture of puff pastry.

Commonly carbohydrate-based fat replacers are available in microparticle form which makes them readily dispersed in the matrices of bakery products. The most common forms of fat replacers are:

- Cellulose- and fibre-based derivatives from a range of sources. Insoluble and soluble fibres may be present, and they are derived from a wide range of grains and legumes.
- Maltodextrins derived from grains, potato, and tapioca.
- Modified starches derived from a number of plant sources.
- Gums such as guar, locust bean, xanthan.
- Polydextrose (e.g. Litesse™) based on a water-soluble polymer of dextrose with a reduced energy value.
- Polyols used to replace fat because of their plasticising and humectant properties and a lower energy contribution.

6.5.7 Protein-Based Replacers

Egg, milk or whey proteins sometimes form the basis of protein-based fat replacers. They may be used alone or in conjunction with a carbohydrate-based fat replacer. While these fat replacers have found use in the liquid or semi-solid foods, their value is limited in bakery products because they are not likely to contribute to structure formation. In addition to the reduction in recipe fat, some contribution to reducing product energy density may be achieved.

6.5.8 Fat/Lipid-Based Replacers

These fat-replacers include those lipid-based ingredients which have lower energy value than fat. This result is achieved by modifying the structure of the lipid (often by esterification) such that its absorption in the human digestive system is reduced. Such materials aid in bulking-out the product. The potential for using such replacers has so far, been limited in bakery products.

6.5.9 'Fat-Free'

While a strict definition of fat-free would be that the food contains no fat, commonly there will be a very low level of fat allowed; for example, in the EU the foods containing <0.5 g fat per 100 g of product may be called fat-free. Many bakery ingredients contain low levels of lipids which will assay as fat with common analytical methods; for example, wheat flour may contain around 1% lipid. Thus, to devise a fat-free bakery product it will be necessary to carefully choose raw materials containing relatively low levels of intrinsic fat (i.e. fat which cannot be removed without affecting the functionality of the raw material) and there would have to be no added recipe fat. Many of the fat replacers identified above are used in conjunction with recipe fat and thus only deliver a partial replacement. There is no doubt that the formulation of bakery products to be fat-free represents a significant technical challenge.

6.6 Reducing Sugar and Changing Sugar Type

While the most obvious role for the addition of sugars to bakery product recipes is to deliver sweetness, there are many other roles that are important; these include contributions to crust colour formation and Maillard browning (also part of product flavour), and the formation of the required product structures and textures. There are also significant contributions to lengthening product sensory shelf-life by reducing the rate at which products stale and to the control of product water activity which in turn, have major impacts on product microbial shelf-life (Cauvain and Young 2008). The many and varied roles of sugars represent major challenges when considering reformulations with respect to product nutrition and the approaches to product development will not necessarily translate readily from one sub-group of bakery products to another. Overall, recipe sugar reduction in many bakery products will involve overcoming a number of significant challenges if product characteristics are to be maintained at, or close to their 'typical' appearance and texture.

6.6.1 Recipe Sugar Reduction

A traditionally held view has been that the addition of sugar (usually sucrose or dextrose) to fermented products is necessary in order to maintain fermentation. This consideration requires qualification in order to understand the opportunities for new product development with reduced sugar levels in fermented product recipes. Wheat flours commonly contain low levels of fermentable sugars and the action of *alpha*-amylase on damaged starch in the flour delivers additional sugar for fermentation (Cauvain 2015). This means that in breadmaking processes where total fermentation times are short, the addition of recipe sugar is seldom necessary to support the fermentation periods employed. This explains why in many parts of the world bread recipes do not contain added sugar. There is a further point to be noted, namely that fermentation in dough depends on the functionality of the bakers' yeast employed. Sucrose, the most commonly used recipe sugar in bread recipes (as discussed earlier), has to be broken down by the enzyme system in the yeast before it can be used for the production of carbon dioxide. In fact, the addition of sucrose to bread dough may actually limit carbon dioxide gas production, especially in the early stages of fermentation, as illustrated in Figure 6.8. In time the bakers' yeast in the dough can adapt to the addition of a disaccharide like sucrose, or an osmo-tolerant yeast strain may be used (Cauvain 2015). The type of sugar available has an influence on the rate at which carbon dioxide gas is produced by yeast fermentation. Most sugars are fermentable by bakers' yeast but changing types has inevitable consequences for manufacturing practices where fermentation times are important. Thus, it would appear that sugar reduction in bread recipes is not only possible but may have technological and cost advantages,

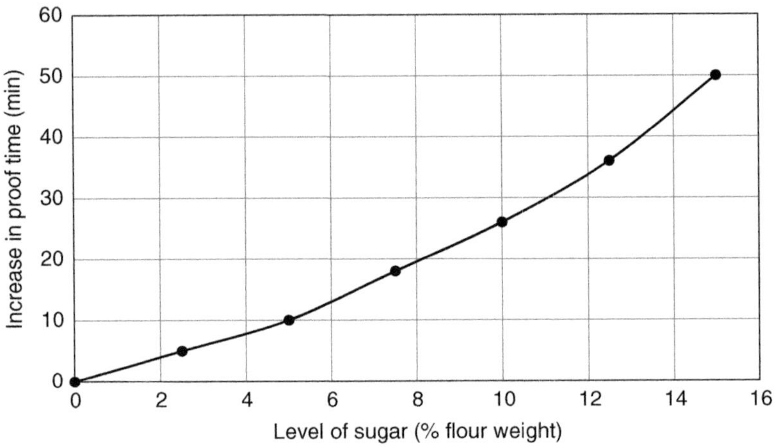

Figure 6.8 Impact of sucrose addition on bread dough fermentation.

not least because it is common with recipe sugar additions to have higher levels of recipe yeast in order to ensure that processing times (e.g. proof) are kept conveniently short. However, in products and processes where recipe sugar has been an intrinsic part of traditional bread and fermented products, lowering recipe sugar levels not only reduces product sweetness but allows other flavours present to become more apparent.

The opportunities associated with sugar reduction in other bakery product sub-groups are potentiality more limited than is the case with fermented products, because of the major contributions that sugars make to final product and textural character. The role of sugar (sucrose) in cake making where its level has to be balanced with the moisture content in order to deliver specific cake qualities is well known (Cauvain and Young 2008; Cauvain 2017). The interaction between the sugar (sucrose) solution in the batter with wheat starch is crucial and this limits opportunities for a simple reduction in sugar level (as noted above). In addition to the loss of structural control associated with sugar, there will be changes in crust colour, shelf-life, and product sweetness. In cake making the bulking effect of sugar is important since recipe sugar reductions inevitably lead to increases in the fat proportion in the final product and with that increase of course, comes an increase in product energy density.

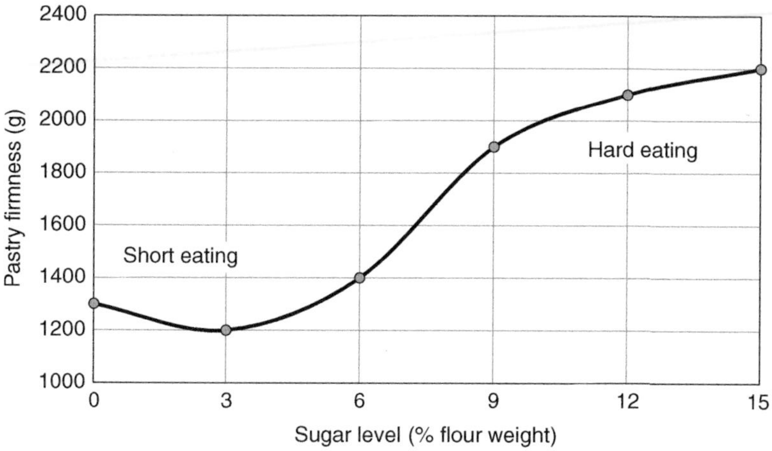

Figure 6.9 Impact of sugar reduction on puff pastry texture.

In biscuits and cookies the level of recipe sugar varies significantly. In cookie products reductions in sugar will lead to significantly less flow during baking and may also result in the loss of 'traditional' surface characteristics; for example, a loss of surface cracking on ginger nut cookies (Cauvain 2017), and reductions in the 'crunchy' eating qualities of such products. Laminated pastry texture is also affected by changes in sugar as illustrated in Figure 6.9; in this case reductions in recipe sugar level tending to deliver a more tender eating texture and greater flakiness.

6.6.2 Changing Sugar Type

It is common among many consumers to equate sugar with sucrose and to a certain extent, refined or white forms of sucrose. This perception can potentially lead to misconceptions when reformulation to reduce product sugar levels is carried out. In terms of energy contributions all sugars are considered equal, though as noted above, there have been arguments put forward that when it comes to the breakdown of sugars in the human digestive system not all sugars are equal. This may be the case, but when it comes to food analyses and labelling declarations, the more common practice is to provide data on the sum total of the different sugars present in the product. Thus, the case for replacing sucrose with another type of sugar and making claims for sugar reduction, is not scientifically nor legislatively established.

While replacing sucrose with another form of sugar may not affect the energy density in a bakery product, it will most certainly affect many other product characteristics. Perhaps the best well-known effect will be on product sweetness. In Table 6.4 the relative sweetness values of some common sugars are compared with that of sucrose. Any losses in sweetness (but not structural functionality) which may occur when sugar type is changed, may be compensated for by the addition of a high intensity sweetener (see Table 6.5). A particular

Table 6.4 Relative sweetness of common sugar types.

Sugar type	Sweetness impact compared with sucrose (= 100), on a weight for weight basis
Dextrose (glucose solids)	~75
Fructose	175
High fructose corn syrup	100–160 depending on type
Maltose	40
Malt syrups	~30
Lactose	20
Corn syrups (depends on DE)	40–80 with increasing DE
Honey	95–100
Molasses	70–70
Brown sugars	85–90

Table 6.5 Common forms of high-intensity sweeteners.

High intensity sweetener	Sweetness impact compared with sucrose (= 1), weight for weight
Acesulfame K	200
Aspartame	200
Sodium cyclamate	30
Sodium saccharin	300
Sucralose	600
Stevia	200–300

concern with high-intensity sweeteners is the potential for breakdown with the high temperatures and long baking times associated with bakery products, which may limit their contribution to product sweetness. While some sweeteners have a sodium component to their composition, their level of use in any baked product recipe is probably too low to have any impact on the overall sodium levels in baked products. For more information on high-intensity sweeteners, readers are referred elsewhere (Nelson 2000).

The functional contribution of sucrose to the formation of cake structures has already been noted. The main impact is related to the concentration of sucrose in the liquid phase of the batter which influences the gelatinisation temperature of the wheat starch in the recipe. Replacing sucrose with other types of sugar inevitably leads to changes in the influence on starch gelatinisation and, in turn, on the formation of product structure. For example, replacing sucrose with dextrose leads to earlier gelatinisation of the starch and, in turn, to a restriction of product volume, changes in cake shape, often along with darkening of the external crust and internal crumb colours; an example of such an effect when dextrose is used is illustrated in Figure 6.10. Once the cake crust sets it is permeable and carbon dioxide produced in the core of the batter after crust setting is readily lost; the ultimate effect is similar to cake recipes baked with low levels of chemical aerating agents (Cauvain 2017). Replacement of sucrose with other sugars (and polyhydric alcohols) may also lead to an uneven crumb colour, typically showing as progressive darkening towards the base of large cakes (Cauvain and Young 2006). Even a partial replacement of sucrose with

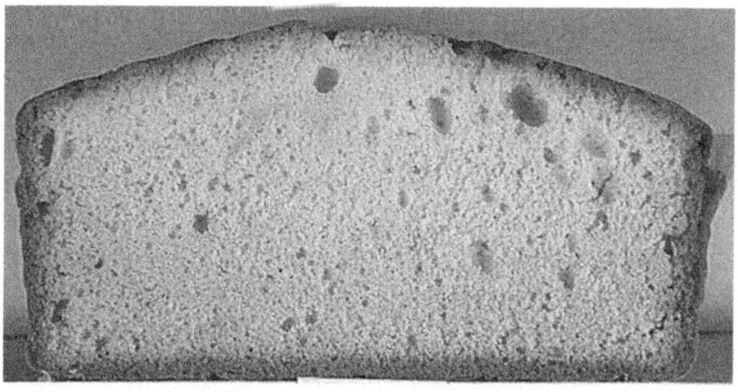

Figure 6.10 Replacement of sucrose with dextrose in cake (cf standard cake – Figure 6.5 a).

another sugar can lead to negative changes in cake quality. In cookies and pastries the replacement of sucrose with other sugars often has a textural impact in addition to changes in sweetness and colour. The spread and texture of many cookies are controlled by the particle size of the sugar (sucrose) (Cauvain 2016) and partial replacement of sucrose with other sugars can affect a number of cookie quality characteristics.

6.6.3 Alternatives to Sugars

Replacers for sugars fall into two broad categories; intense sweeteners and polyols. The introduction of intense sweeteners into bakery products tends to be limited, not least because while it is relatively easy to deliver a sweet taste with such ingredients, their levels of addition are very low. Thus, in a bakery product the bulk and functional effects of sugars will be entirely missing. There are also some technical concerns about the ability of some intense sweeteners to remain unaffected by the high baking temperatures and long times; often this means the delivery of a lower level of sweetness than would be the case for soft drinks and in a few cases, there may be adverse flavour development as a result of breakdown reactions in the baking process itself. Many polyols are hygroscopic, that is they readily absorb water, and in some cases high levels of polyols in a recipe may induce stickiness on the product surface. Such effects are often seen with cake products and will cause the crust to stick to the overwrapping film.

Polyols or sugar alcohols are less sweet than many sugars and tend to deliver lower energy values on a weight for weight basis. Thus, they are more suited to being used as sugar replacers, though their functionality and ability to deliver specific baked product structures is far from that achieved by sugars. Some common polyols and sugar alcohols are listed in Table 6.6, along with some of their key properties. Polyols are non-fermentable, a factor which must be taken into account when replacing sugars in bread production. They also change the gelatinisation character of wheat starch and thus the formation of cake structures (e.g. shape). Polyols break down during prolonged heating and this tends to lead to discolouration in the crumb of the final cake; there may also be adverse changes in product crust colour and appearance. The levels at which polyols may be present in food formulae may be subjected to legislative restriction because of potential negative digestive effects. For example, some polyols are known to

Table 6.6 Common polyols and sugar alcohols.

Polyol	Source	Energy density (kcal g^{-1})	Approximate sweetness compared with sucrose (= 100)
Sorbitol	Polyhydroxy alcohol derived from dextrose	2.6	50–70
Xylitol	Derived from fermented plant pulp	2.4	100
Maltitol	Starch transposed to maltose syrup and hydrogenated	2.1	75
Isomalt	Derived from sugar beet	2.0	45–65
Lactitol	Derived from lactose	2.0	30–40
Mannitol	Derived from corn starch	1.6	50–70
Eryhritol	Derived from corn starch	0.2	60–80
Hydrogenated starch hydrolysates	Derived from corn starch	3.0	25–50

induce a laxative effect in the bowel. The maximum levels of such polyols will be specified in legislation and commonly related to daily intakes, with levels recommended for children being significantly lower than that for adults; readers are advised to check local legislation with respect to the use of polyols.

6.6.4 'Sugar-Free', No Added Sugar and No Refined Sugar

In the past the term sugar-free has commonly become associated with the removal of recipe sucrose and the subsequent health links with a reduction of dental caries, or with the manufacture of sugar-free products for diabetics. While not underestimating the importance of sucrose- and sugar-free products in either of the previous contexts, it is not the primary purpose of this work to cover such issues in detail. Within the context of this work, the descriptors used for this section are considered in relation to their contribution to energy density and general, rather than specific, contributions to the diet (for more relevant material see Goran et al. 2015). As discussed above, in most bakery products the removal of sucrose and its replacement with other sugars does not affect the energy density of the product and in labelling terms, other sugars will contribute to the analytical measurement of total sugars. The term sugar-free is therefore difficult, if not impossible, to apply to bakery products and often one sees the descriptor 'no added' sugar, again principally being applied to recipes which contain no added sucrose. Another descriptor which has been applied to some food products has been that of 'no refined sugars'. Again, this is aimed primarily at sucrose and white or 'refined' forms of sucrose. There is no evidence to show that non-refined sugars change to the contribution of energy density of bakery products, unless that is a weight for weight replacement does not contribute the same physical quantity of sugar, i.e. there are other materials present in the non-refined sugar. The position for sugar replacers in this context has been discussed above.

6.7 Reducing Energy (Calories)

The challenges associated with reformulation in order to develop bakery products which have a reduction in energy density have been introduced above, and it is clear that in order to deliver a significant energy reduction it will be necessary to introduce ingredients into the recipe which have lower energy values than the commonly used macronutrients. Water contributes no kilojoules to a bakery formula, but the problems associated with raising recipe and product moisture contents have been highlighted above, not least of which is the potential shortening of microbial-free shelf-life. Few permitted food ingredients have truly low energy values per unit weight and those that do, typically lack the complete functionality of the ingredient(s) that they are 'replacing'. As there are no unique low energy ingredient replacers which substantially exhibit the same functionality of the ingredients they purport to replace, it is necessary to take a holistic view in the development of energy-reduced bakery products. Reformulation for reduced-energy products will thus require the introduction of a number of different ingredients, each potentially making a small, but important contribution to energy reduction in the final product (Barker and Cauvain 1994). This holistic approach may also mitigate some of the negative functional and sensory effects when large quantity replacements are affected with some ingredients (e.g. see discussion on polyols above).

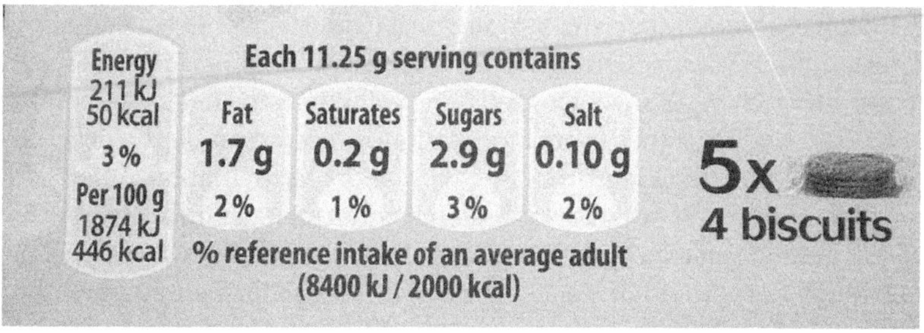

Figure 6.11 Example of energy declaration per serving for a breakfast biscuit.

While not strictly a means of reduced the energy density of the final products, there has been a trend in many markets to reduce the portion size of the final product. This is often associated with claims related to the number of kilojoules per unit or serving (see Figure 6.11). This means that if the consumer simply eats the same number of product units, then the total energy intake will be reduced. The reduction of product portion size has been encouraged as part of anti-obesity strategies by many government agencies and as part of a 'responsible' industry approach. Such approaches may well be combined with a true reduction in product energy density through reformulation rather than size alone.

6.8 Reducing Salt (Sodium)

In some parts of the world (e.g. the UK) the reduction of salt has been practised for over 20 years, while in others it is in its early stages of implementation. There are two broad strategies which may be employed; one is to reduce the overall level of salt (sodium chloride) in a product and the other to 'replace' the salt with an alternative. The particular strategies employed for reducing salt (or sodium) will vary according to the functional properties of salt in the different bakery product subgroups (Cauvain 2007). In bread and other fermented products, by far the most common approach has been to reduce the level of recipe salt, usually on a gradual basis, with target reductions being set on a voluntary or regulatory basis. The technological changes required to cope with reduced salt bread levels in bread are most commonly those associated with the control of fermentation and compensation for changes in dough rheology, especially in larger-scale industrial bread production. As salt inhibits yeast activity (Cauvain 2015), a reduction in salt level may require that changes in yeast levels, or fermentation times and conditions (e.g. temperature), or a combination of both may be required. In the case of breadmaking processes with short fermentation times (i.e. processes which do not allow the dough to ferment in bulk before it is divided, often referred to as 'no-time doughs'), changes in yeast level in the dough are commonly small because the overall fermentation period is short and confined to the stage commonly referred by bakers as proof (or final proof). Nevertheless, the balance between salt and yeast level remains important and extends to the final burst of gas production in the early stages of the baking process where, if excess gas production occurs, it may contribute to loss of product shape and the formation of unwanted holes in bread crumb (BakeTran 2012b).

The situation with regard to the impact of reduced salt levels on dough rheology and handling is more complex. It is commonly considered that salt, because of its ability to readily combine with water, contributes to dough development and with reduced salt levels it is generally considered that the hydration of wheat flour proteins, and the manner in which the subsequent gluten network is adversely affected (Belz et al. 2012). One of the negative impacts of reducing recipe salt levels is an increase in dough stickiness, as shown by Cauvain (2015). While sticky doughs can be readily accommodated when moulding dough by hand (with the use of a little extra 'dusting' flour), the mechanical shear induced by mechanical moulding equipment in industrial bread production can lead to particular problems, including loss of yield and plant stoppages. Some modification of plant operation may need to be introduced in order to cope with dough stickiness arising from a reduction in salt level. This may include the introduction of dusting flour (not popular in many industrial bakeries), the use of air blowers to 'dry' the dough surface (Cauvain 2015), or the adoption of alternative dough moulding practices. Ultimately the reduction in recipe salt level does yield doughs which are more sensitive in large-scale production and there is an increased need for improved process control as a result of the change.

The impact of reducing recipe salt on bread flavour is the area of greatest concern to bakers, not least because the loss of flavour may lead to lower bread consumption and the loss of other nutritional benefits for consumers (e.g. lower calcium and fibre intakes). As shown by the UK experience, consumers' palates can indeed be re-educated to lower salt levels in bread, but the other contributors to bread flavour, particularly from fermentation, are more subtle and have a lesser impact on the perception of bread quality. The principles associated with producing acidic flavours in bread as the result of fermentation are well known (see for example, Gobbetti and Ganzle 2013) but not all consumers around the world welcome the astringent flavour that sour dough production yields in bread.

A number of salt (sodium chloride) alternatives have been suggested. Potassium chloride may be used as a partial replacement for sodium chloride but unfortunately, as the overall level of sodium chloride falls in bread, so does the proportion of it that can be replaced with the potassium salt before the bitterness associated with latter become evident (Kilcast and den Ridder 2007). Partial replacement of sodium chloride with magnesium or calcium chlorides (Charlton et al. 2007) may also be used (provided their use is permitted), but again levels of substitution are limited. In all cases the impact of all such alternatives on dough development differs from that of the sodium chloride.

The challenge for reducing salt in other sub-groups of bakery products is perhaps greater than that for bread. This is not because recipe salt levels are high in such products, indeed typically they are lower in cakes than in bread. The problem lies with those products which rely on chemical aeration since many baking powders contain high levels of sodium compounds which when measured analytically, are converted to salt equivalents under most legislation or labelling requirements around the world (the reasons for this approach have been discussed above). The sodium may be associated with both the acid and base components in baking powders. While there are many options for constructing baking powders without or with low levels of sodium-based materials, such changes can have a significant impact on the flavour of the final product. The residual salts remaining from a baking powder reaction have distinctive flavours in the baked product, depending on the nature of the composition of compounds employed and this too must be taken into account when reducing sources of sodium in chemically aerated products.

Reducing recipe sodium levels or substituting sodium in the acid or base will require significant adjustment to the composition of the baking powder. One of the greatest challenges associated with reducing the sodium levels in chemically-raised bakery products, is the potential change in the functionality of the baking powder. The acid and base levels in a baking powder are not only balanced to deliver the required level of carbon dioxide gas in a matrix, but also to optimise the time of release of the gas to exert the greatest effect in terms of product structure; this is commonly referred to as the 'rate of reaction' (Cauvain 2017). The different acids which may be used as part of the leavening system have very different rates of reaction and indeed, even the same acid may be available in different forms (usually particle size), each of which will have a different rate of reaction.

While there are a number of baking acids which may be used to generate the necessary carbon dioxide from the baking powder mix, it is perhaps the replacement of the sodium bicarbonate which can be the most difficult to achieve. Potassium bicarbonate, potassium carbonate, ammonium bicarbonate and calcium carbonate, may all be used as alternative sources of the carbon dioxide necessary for chemical leavening. Each alternative will require a rebalancing of the acid to carbonate source levels and as with the different leavening acids, the rates and conditions of reaction for each of the alternative carbon dioxide sources vary. The choice of alternative to sodium bicarbonate will also influence the flavour of the residual salts which may in turn, influence consumer acceptability. Readers involved in seeking low sodium baking powders are advised to consult with specialist suppliers of leavening agents.

6.9 Increasing Dietary Fibre

The introduction of increased fibre into bakery products has a long history, at least as far as bread is concerned. Wholemeal flour represents a most obvious way of increasing fibre in bakery products but while it has been readily accepted in bread, at least by some consumer groups, fibre-enrichment is less prevalent in other bakery products. In part, this is because the drier and rougher mouthfeel arising from the presence of some types of fibre particles (e.g. wheat bran) in bread is even less acceptable in many other bakery product sub-groups, such as pastries. In addition to the impact of bran on product eating quality, the presence of bran particles often has negative impacts on product structure and visual appearance which are not consistent with consumer expectations for some bakery products.

There are many sources of dietary fibre which may be used in the manufacture of bakery products. Some do not have the same negative physical impacts imparted by wheat bran, though each source has its own challenges when introduced into bakery products. A common property of the various forms of fibre is their ability to hold water and so it is usually a requirement to increase recipe water levels to restore dough or batter rheology to normal processing levels. This may precipitate further recipe or process changes with those products in which low moisture is a key final product characteristic (e.g. crackers and cookies), or where a higher final moisture content would compromise product shelf-life (e.g. cakes).

Choosing an ingredient for the specific purpose of increasing dietary fibre in a bakery product will depend on many factors. The consumer acceptability of the raw material on the product listing is amongst the most important. All sources of dietary fibre will be natural, though the individual source may not be 'common' to consumers. This situation often applies to dietary fibre sourced as by-products of other raw material processing, e.g. fruit pulps (Figuerola et al. 2005); while apple fibre may be seen as an acceptable ingredient with cakes, it may be less so with chocolate cookies. A practical issue for many proposed sources of dietary fibre is the sufficiency of supply, especially if they are a by-product of some other food processing environment. The choice of dietary fibre source will be judged against the purpose of its addition. If the intention is to meet specific dietary claims this will dictate, to some extent, its level of addition. Some of the practical and quality problems associated with dietary fibre addition have been noted above. Such issues may obviate the use of some sources, especially those with lower concentrations of dietary fibre. Other practical problems may be related to the colour and particle size of the dietary fibre source as these will have profound impacts on product appearance, texture, and eating qualities, all of which are key to consumer product acceptance.

6.10 Fortification for Health Benefits

The practices and opportunities for introducing health benefits via fortification of raw materials and bakery products have been discussed above. Traditionally many of the routes to fortification in bakery products are based on introducing health benefits via the flour, because flour is by far the most commonly used ingredient in baking. Fortification of flours does not usually come with particular production or technical challenges in the manufacture of baked foodstuff. More recently the introduction of potential health benefits has spread to other raw materials which may be used in baking, for example vitamin D via yeast and iodine in salt (see Chapter 3).

There are numerous, naturally occurring raw materials which may be considered as sources of health benefits in bakery products. Some may already be permitted and the numbers continue to increase. Unlike flour fortification approaches, the addition of such materials is not without its challenges. These may be broadly grouped into two broad categories; technological functionality and heat stability. While many raw materials may be rich, natural sources of vitamins and minerals with defined health benefits for humans, they may be associated with other components which can have negative impacts on doughs, batters, and baked products. One area which is often of concern, is associated with the introduction of strong flavours, sometimes from the raw material itself, or through reactions with other recipe ingredients, or which develop during processing. The oven baking process is often associated with the development of unwanted or atypical flavours as the combination of high temperatures and often long baking times can lead to the degradation of raw material components.

The high temperatures in the oven and associated long baking times may lead to degradation of some of the components added in the first instance to deliver health benefits. The presence of high water levels in dough and batters can often exacerbate the degradation of sources of health befits. Minerals are heat stable but the same cannot be said for vitamins, and often their survival into the finished product is questionable. Thus, while fortification of baked goods recipes is rightly viewed as an opportunity for conferring health benefits to consumers, its practice is not entirely without its challenges.

6.11 Conclusions

There are many opportunities for improving the health and nutritional profiles of a range of baked products. The fortification of wheat flour has long been practised and presents no particular production or technical challenges. Increasing the fibre content of bread and fermented products using wholemeal flours, seeds, and other raw materials high in dietary fibre is now common practice. However, higher fibre versions of cakes, cookies and pastries are less common and the potential negative effects of fibre-rich raw materials on product texture need to be overcome before higher fibre versions of such products may become common place. The structural impact of fibre-rich raw material will vary according to the source of the fibre and nature of the material.

The opportunities for replacing or reducing fat and sugar in bakery products depend on the sub-group and geographical location being considered. Both fat and sugar make significant contributions to product structure formation as well as texture and flavour. The successful reduction of recipe fat and sugar requires a thorough understanding of the different roles that these ingredients play in the manufacture of different bakery product sub-groups. Fat and sugar replacers are offered in the market place but none are able to deliver the required functionality on a one-to-one basis. In practice the reduction of recipe fat and sugar levels is likely to require multiple formulation changes, complemented by processing changes, or the introduction of new technologies.

References

BakeTran (2012a) A guide to the effects of the main ingredients used in cake and sponge recipes. *Chorleywood Bookshelf Monograph No. 3.* www.baketran.com/

BakeTran (2012b) Unwanted holes in bread: Why they form and how to limit them. *Chorleywood Bookshelf Monograph No. 1.* www.baketran.com/

BakeTran (2017) Technology of laminated products. *Chorleywood Bookshelf Monograph No. 4.* www.baketran.com/

Barker, P. and Cauvain, S.P. (1994). Fat and calorie-modified bakery products. In: *International. Food Ingredients*, vol. 1, 19–24.

Belz, M.C.E., Ryan, L.A.M., and Arendt, E.K. (2012). The impact of salt reduction in bread: a review. *Critical Reviews in Food Science and Nutrition* 52 (6): 514–524.

Brooker, B.E. (1996). The role of fat in the stabilisation of gas cells in bread dough. *Journal of Cereal Science* 24 (3): 187–198.

Cauvain, S.P. (2007). Reducing salt in bread and other bakery products. In: *Reducing Salt in Foods* (ed. D. Kilcast and F. Angus), 283–295. Cambridge, UK: Woodhead Publishing.

Cauvain, S.P. (2015). *Technology of Breadmaking*, 3e. Cham Heidelberg, Switzerland: Springer.

Cauvain, S.P. (2016). Cookies, biscuits and crackers: formulation, processing and characteristics. In: *Encyclopedia of Food Grains*, 2e (ed. C. Wrigley, H. Corke, K. Seetharaman and J. Faubion), 37–43. Oxford, UK: Academic Press.

Cauvain, S.P. (2017). *Baking Problems Solved*, 2e. Duxford, UK: Woodhead Publishing.

Cauvain, S.P. and Young, L.S. (2006). *Baked Products: Science, Technology and Practice*. Oxford, UK: Blackwell Publishing.

Cauvain, S.P. and Young, L.S. (2008). *Bakery Food Manufacture and Quality*, 2e. Oxford, UK: Wiley-Blackwell.

Charlton, K.E., MacGregor, E., Vorster, N.H. et al. (2007). Partial replacement of NaCl can be achieved with potassium, calcium and magnesium salts in brown bread. *International Journal of Food Sciences and Nutrition* 58 (7): 508–521.

Figuerola, F., Hurtado, M.L., Estevez, A.M. et al. (2005). Fibre concentrates from apple pomace and citrus peel as potential fibre sources for food enrichment. *Food Chemistry* 91 (3): 395–401.

Gobbetti, M. and Ganzle, M. (2013). *Handbook on Sourdough Biotechnology*. New York: Springer Science+Business Media.

Goran, M.I., Tappy, L., and Le, K.-A. (2015). *Dietary Sugars and Health*. Boca Raton, FL: CRC Press.

Kilcast, D. and den Ridder, C. (2007). Sensory issues in reducing salt in food products. In: *Reducing Salt in Foods: Practical Strategies* (ed. D. Kilcast and F. Angus), 201–220. Cambridge, UK: Woodhead Publishing.

Kornbrust, B.A., Forman, T., and Mateeva, I. (2012). Application of enzymes in breadmaking. In: *Breadmaking: Improving Quality*, 2e (ed. S.P. Cauvain). Cambridge, UK: Woodhead Publishing.

Nelson, A.L. (2000). *Sweeteners: Alternative*. St. Paul, MN: Eagan Press.

Whitehurst, R.J. (2004). *Emulsifiers in Food Technology*. Oxford, UK: Blackwell Publishing.

Wickramarachchi, K.S., Sissons, M.J., and Cauvain, S.P. (2015). Puff pastry and trends in fat reduction: an update. *International Journal of Food Science and Technology* 50: 1065–1075.

7

Approaches to Development of Nutritionally Enhanced Bakery Products

7.1 Introduction

The necessity for delivering nutritionally enhanced bakery products with sensory properties that will be accepted by consumers has been already been highlighted. Acceptable sensory properties and shelf-life remain critical deliverables for commercially successful products. As noted above, the development of nutritionally enhanced bakery products is not without its challenges, most of which centre on the manner in which product structures are formed in a complex series of ingredient, recipe and process interactions, many of which have been defined for 'conventional' bakery products in empirical terms by bakers over many years. In setting out to develop nutritionally baked products, developers are faced with a number of challenges which at best lie at the limits of conventional recipe construction and in many cases, beyond the normal boundaries of bakery product manufacture. In moving beyond the boundaries of conventional bakery product recipe construction, product developers need to consider the most appropriate approaches to use in the development process. When operating outside of traditional paradigms for bakery products, the default position tends to be to undertake a series of trial-and-error developments, with exploration of those avenues which show greatest promise. This can be a slow, costly, and high-risk strategy, not least when development time constraints may be in place. There are a wide range of techniques which may be applied to improve the efficiency and potential success of the product development approach and this chapter will consider some of these.

Baking Technology and Nutrition: Towards a Healthier World, First Edition.
Stanley P. Cauvain and Rosie H. Clark.

7.2 Empirical Rules and Product Development

In the case of many types of bakery products, it is common practice for bakers to construct recipes with functional ingredient quantities based on the flour weight in the recipe. Typically, the recipe description will therefore be expressed in terms of bakers' percent; an example is shown in Table 7.1 where the flour weight is expressed as 100 and the quantities of all other ingredients are shown relative to that number. This approach contrasts with the other common methods of expressing ingredient weights in recipes as a percentage of the total mass; i.e. a proportion of a total of 100. There is no right or wrong way of constructing bakery product recipes, though the traditional bakers' percentage does offer a practical method for understanding the consequences of manipulating ingredient levels in recipes.

As noted above, many empirical rules underpin the manufacture of bakery products. Some of these empirical rules have been identified and published in the past, with relatively little updating. The approaches used with these empirical rulesets are commonly based on the functionality and contribution of specific ingredients to final product quality. In a few cases these empirical rules have been broadly quantified (Bent 1997). The nature of the rules varies with the different subgroups of bakery products. A major problem with empirical rules is

Table 7.1 Cake recipe expressed in Bakers' percentage.

Ingredient	Bakers' %	Batter %
Flour	100	26.60
Margarine	60	15.96
Sugar	90	23.94
Skimmed milk powder	4	1.06
Whole egg	60	15.96
Baking powder	2	0.53
Water	30	7.98
Dried fruit	30	7.98
Total	376	100.00

that there is a prerequisite for a defined final product quality. This has certainly been the case with the historical rules which have been applied to the structure of cake recipes for the production of traditional cake forms, such as Madeira (Thomas Hedley 1958), pound, and sponge cakes. While such rules of cake recipe balance are aimed at enabling bakers to produce a 'prefect' cake, they refer to a range of acceptable ingredient levels rather than prescriptive levels. This does at least allow bakers a degree of individuality in the manufacture of their cakes which in part, explains why cakes with a common descriptor (e.g. Madeira) do not all have the same appearance, texture, and taste. There are also potential quality impacts from processing variations.

While empirical baking rules were designed to help bakers avoid quality defects in their products, the information that they enshrine does have some value for use in the context of new product development. In many ways product development can be likened to problem-solving, in the sense that the developer is seeking to modify the characteristics of the final product. When solving a problem, the bakery technologist is seeking to rectify a quality defect while in the development process the aim is to introduce particular quality characteristics which are absent from the starting product. By way of example two cakes are illustrated in Figure 7.1. It is clear that amongst other features that the profiles of the two products are distinctly different with one having a flat top and the other a peaked shape. If the flat surface was the accepted standard for the product concerned, then the peaked shape would be seen as a quality defect and by using the empirical rules of recipe balance, reformulation would be used to adjust the product shape and any other negative quality aspects. As noted above, the same empirical rules that were used to solve a quality problem could be used for product development. In this scenario the peaked cake profile could be the accepted standard while the development required could be to make products with a flat profile. Cauvain (2017a) suggested such a duality for information associated with problem-solving and new product development.

There have been attempts to enshrine problem-solving and baking recipe balance approaches within computer-based knowledge systems (Young 1995, 1996, 2007; Young et al. 1998). In the context of new product development, the approach was to allow users to develop their knowledge and skills at the computer by posing a series of 'what if?' questions. The computer program would deliver answers based on the examination of specific rule bases which encapsulated both

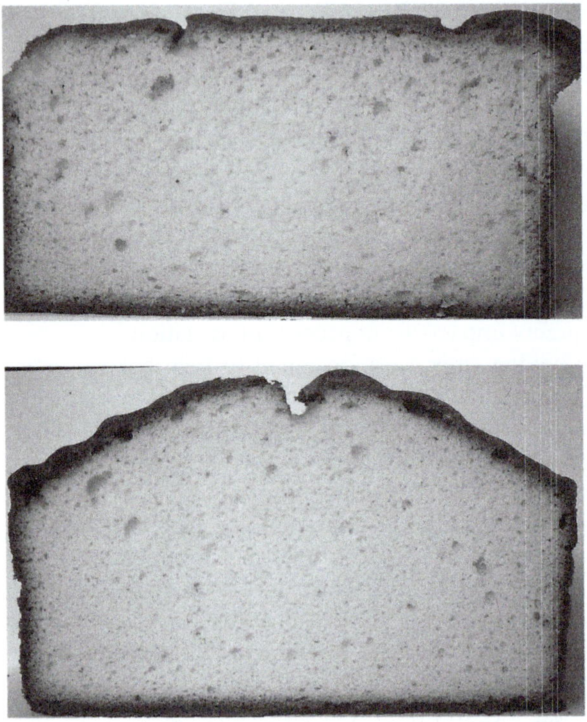

Figure 7.1 Examples of cake profiles.

interactions between recipe ingredients (similar to those historically described for recipe construction) and most importantly, the interaction of the recipe with the processing methods applied in the manufacture of the chosen bakery products. A number of commercially available computer-based systems were developed which could be applied to different aspects of bakery production at a time when computing power and computer graphics were modest by comparison those available today. Unfortunately, the developments were discontinued and none of the systems are available commercially today.

7.3 Mathematics and Product Development

There is a wide range of mathematical techniques which may be used for establishing mathematical models to aid product development; these may be considered as the quantitative equivalent of the empirical approach described briefly above. In order to establish rules of a mathematical nature it is necessary to have access to relevant data. Commonly such data will be derived from objective studies related to the ingredients, recipes and processes which apply to the manufacture of bakery products. There are few instances of data-based models being established in the bakery product manufacturing environment, not least because those studies which are available are highly specific to a particular product area or process, and often related to the optimisation of existing product types rather than the development of new products. The position may be illustrated by looking at the bakery products map outlined in Figure 2.1 (page 24). Here the boundaries of recipe construction are defined in two dimensions based on three ingredients, flour, sugar and fat. It can be argued that 'normal' products cannot exist outside of these boundaries, though it can equally be argued that the 'empty' spaces are where new products may be found, not least in the context of this work for nutritionally enhanced bakery products.

A key step in developing information that permits the creation of new models for bakery products is the gathering and analysis of relevant data. Of critical importance in developing new mathematical models is the performance of research within a clearly structured plan. In its simplest form the model may be comprise a series of databases which can be interrogated by the user; they may be paper-based but today it is more common to use a computer-based system. The knowledge-based programs referred to above represent a form of model which may be described as symbolic that is, not purely based on mathematics and quantitative models may be part of such a system. The water activity calculation and mould-free shelf-life prediction program – Equilibrium Relative Humidity (ERH) CALC™ (Cauvain and Young 2008) – initially developed by the Flour Milling and Baking Research Association (FMBRA), Chorleywood – was an example of how databases and mathematical models could be combined to provide a functional product development tool. In that system ingredients were selected from the database which contained relevant analytical data, and used to construct product recipes, either existing or under development. Within the program it was possible to calculate the product water activity (or ERH) and estimate the minimum mould-free shelf-life. Such tools can be invaluable in product development as they allow individuals to try out many ideas in a short space of time, thus speeding up the product development process. When linked with a nutritional database, such symbolic models are particularly useful for the development of nutritionally enhanced bakery products, as will be further discussed below.

The development of more formal mathematical models is commonly based on applying various statistical analytical techniques to experimental data, most often derived from laboratory or pilot-scale studies. Essential to the successful development of relevant models is the initial experimental design. Too often statistical analysis is applied to data without due consideration of the objective of the experimental work. There are many techniques available for statistical analysis of experimental data and choosing the most appropriate one depends on the defined purpose of the study and the choice of experimental design. Street (1991) provides a useful summary of statistical techniques and discusses them in the context of problem-solving and the development of new bakery products. There are many examples of relevant baking related studies in the literature, though most are confined to a narrow area of ingredient or baking technology.

The challenge for baking has been and to some extent remains, the nature of baking processes in which there are many complex interactions between ingredients and processes. An old axiom when performing experiments is to change only one thing at a time in the study. In baking one could argue that this is impossible because of the ingredient–recipe–process interactions. This has made the process of problem-solving in baking complex and equally makes the development of new products challenging. Let us consider a topic encompassed within this work, namely the reduction of salt in bread and fermented products. A reduction in recipe salt level is known to have technological effects on dough development and yeast activity (see above). To reduce the potentially negative impact of lower salt levels on dough development it may be necessary to adjust the level of other recipe ingredients or mixing conditions, or a combination of both. In the case of yeast activity, lower salt levels may result in faster processing times (e.g. shorter final proof) but it may not be possible to accommodate such a change practically in the bakery; additionally shorter processing times may well bring with them negative impacts on dough rheology and final product quality. An alternative to reducing processing times is to reduce recipe yeast level with lower salt levels in order to maintain constant final proof times. However, reduced recipe yeast levels may have a negative impact on oven spring and crumb cell structure. Once again, the challenge for the product developer is how to balance the complex effects that come with what appears to be a relatively simple, single modification to the recipe.

7.4 Visualisation and Simulation Techniques for Product Development

One way in which the complex relationships associated with baking may be modelled is to combine both subjective and objective data using visualisation or simulation techniques. Cauvain and Young (2006) suggested some simple visualisation techniques which could be applied to identifying the direction of change in a product property without necessarily quantifying that change. In one sense bakers have been using such visualisation techniques for many years in that one often sees references to the role of specific bakery ingredients in modifying specific product properties. For example, the role of fat in biscuits and cake is often described in terms of changes in product eating quality. This is commonly along the lines that increasing the recipe fat level delivers a 'shorter' eating quality, and the opposite if fat levels are reduced. To some extent this explains the use of the colloquial term 'shortening' as applied to composite bakery fats. So, a simple approach to considering the reduction of recipe fat levels could be to recognise that a reduction in fat level will result in a less short (less soft or harder) eating quality and to seek to compensate for that directional change in eating quality with some other ingredient, recipe, or process change. Even this approach is not straightforward if we consider, for example, the relation between fat and whole egg in cake recipes. Traditionally fat and egg levels in cakes recipes are 'balanced' because fat delivers a shorter eating quality (i.e. it is a 'tenderiser') while egg delivers a firmer eating quality, largely as a result of the proteins which are present. Thus, in this case a reduction in cake recipe fat level may also require a reduction in egg level in order to restore eating qualities. As always, the challenge is what does the recipe developer use in the place of the 'missing' fat and egg levels which will maintain product acceptability while delivering enhanced nutrition? In the context of current nutritional focus at the time of writing, the proportional increase in recipe sugars would not be seen as acceptable in some circles.

Cauvain and Young (2006) introduced a simple visualisation technique which could be used in both problem-solving (Cauvain 2017a) and product development. The concept was based on the development of 'knowledge trees' and 'knowledge fragments' which seek to summarise key relationships which contribute to particular product qualities in a hierarchical structure. The principle was that the 'knowledge tree' was the high-level summary while the 'knowledge

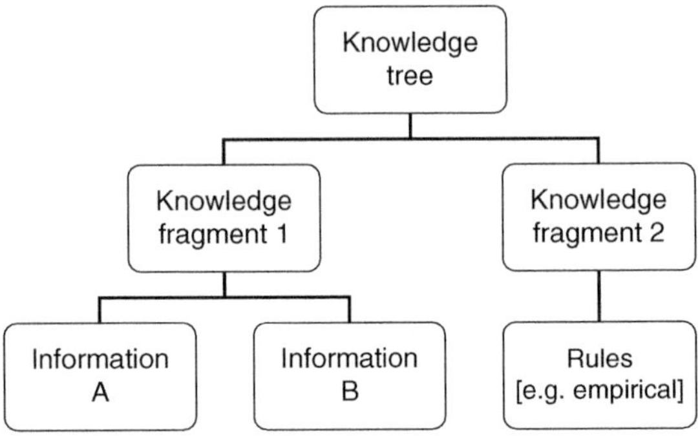

Figure 7.2 Principles of the knowledge tree visualisation approach.

fragment' provided more detail on one of the elements identified in the knowledge tree. The intention was that all the necessary information associated with a knowledge tree could be represented on one page or screen, with each knowledge fragment being related to only one element of the tree. This multi-layered approach could be used for qualitative information, but could also include quantitative information, where available. The principle by which such an approach might work is illustrated in Figure 7.2.

An example of how visualisation using the concepts of knowledge trees and fragments might be used in the product development of nutritionally enhanced bakery products would be appropriate. The nutritional requirement relates to the development of a cake product in which specific claims under EU rules are required for sources of fibre and protein. Compositionally the former requires that the recipe contributes at least 3% of dietary fibre and that in case of the latter at least 12% of the cake should comprise protein (which should also be 12% of the calories). A variety of ingredient sources are available to contribute to these nutritional objectives, but not all may be compatible with the requisite technical functional requirements related to production and product quality. The first step in this development path would be to establish the primary attributes that consumers would want/expect from a typical cake product. The next step would be to take from that list the most critical aspect, in consumer terms, of the expected eating quality for that type of product. Examples of appropriate cake textural attributes terms used by consumers are given in Table 7.2. It should be noted that in this context we have

Table 7.2 Examples of cake textural attributes terms.

Dry
Moist
Crumbly
Hard
Soft
Tender
Short
Dense
Light
Fragile
Tough

made no attempt to define the individual attributes in sensory panel terms; for such purposes readers are referred elsewhere (Meilgaard et al. 2016).

For the purposes of understanding how the knowledge tree approach might be used for the development of a nutritionally enhanced cake based on fibre and protein claims as described above, the consumer perception of final cake moistness (softness) has been chosen for consideration, because it represents a commonly requested and sought property of cake products. Based on this attribute, a knowledge tree can be constructed using those known factors which are likely to contribute to perceived product moistness, and it is illustrated in Figure 7.3. The left-hand leg of the diagram deals with the most obvious contributor to cake moistness, namely the moisture content of the cake; one would anticipate that the more moisture that remains in the cake the greater will be its perceived moistness. This is certainly the case, though with increased cake moisture there is the inevitable restriction of shelf-life, so while a simple increase in recipe water level may be considered, or a reduction in baking losses, there will be important consequences for other quality attributes. In addition to concerns over shelf-life, there would be the possibility of other unwanted changes in product quality with increased recipe water addition, such as the example illustrated in Figure 7.4 which shows how an excess of water in a cake recipe can contribute to the sinking of fruit during baking. Related to moisture content, though not the

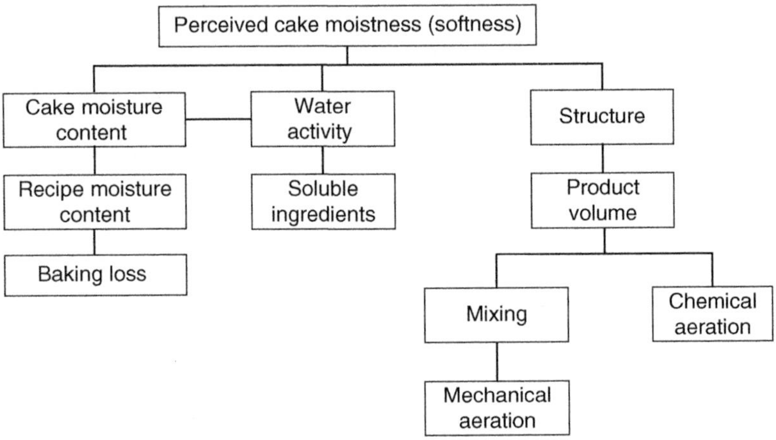

Figure 7.3 Example of a knowledge-tree outlining the factors which affect product moistness.

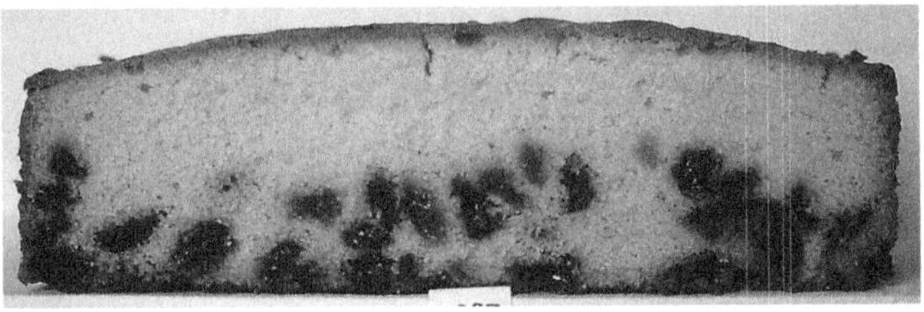

Figure 7.4 Effect of increasing water on fruit cake quality.

same property, is product water activity. Some of the ingredients available for cake making have a profound effect on water activity and shelf-life without their addition completely negating the potential for delivering increased moisture content (Cauvain and Young 2008).

Often the consumer perception of cake 'moistness' is linked with cake softness, a textural property which is affected by a number on non-moisture related factors. Cakes with an increased volume (lower density) are often perceived to be softer and moister to eat. In this case the perception of moistness is a consequence of a change in cake structure. To the right-hand side of the knowledge-tree illustrated in Figure 7.4, is a leg which considers the potential impact of product structure on the perception of moistness (or softness). This shows how changes to the cake structure may be brought about by increasing cake volume, such as by manipulating batter aeration to deliver increased cake volume. There are two broad approaches which may be used; mechanical aeration controlled by mixing conditions and chemical aeration using leavening agents (*BakeTran* 2012). In order to exploit such approaches, it will be necessary to understand in greater detail how to deliver the required benefits without comprising other product attributes. This more detailed examination of a particular option would be carried out by passing through the heading in an individual box in the knowledge tree to an underlying knowledge fragment.

The delivery of more information using knowledge fragments drawn from boxes in a knowledge tree allows ingredients and process components to be considered in more detail. In many cases the information can be linked with the practical consequences of changing process conditions or recipe ingredient levels. An example of a knowledge fragment is illustrated for salt in bread in Figure 7.5. In this example the consequences of using less salt on yeast activity in the dough are noted, with a comment on the practical changes which may be required in the bakery. Below an individual box in the knowledge fragment may be a further layer of qualitative and quantitative information.

7.5 The Role of Product Evaluation in the Development of Nutritionally Enhanced Bakery Products

Given that the sensory properties of nutritionally enhanced bakery products are critical to their acceptance by consumers, it is relevant to briefly consider how such products may be evaluated, especially in terms of texture and eating quality. Readers are referred elsewhere for details of objective techniques related to the evaluation of bakery product characteristics such as volume, shape and colour (Cauvain 2015; 2017b). These properties can be readily assessed with established means and are thus easy to define in new product development terms so that they can be readily included in any new product brief, along with acceptable ranges of values. Product texture, taste and eating qualities, however, are less easy to define with objective measurements for inclusion in a product development briefing and their assessment still tends to be based on sensory assessment using

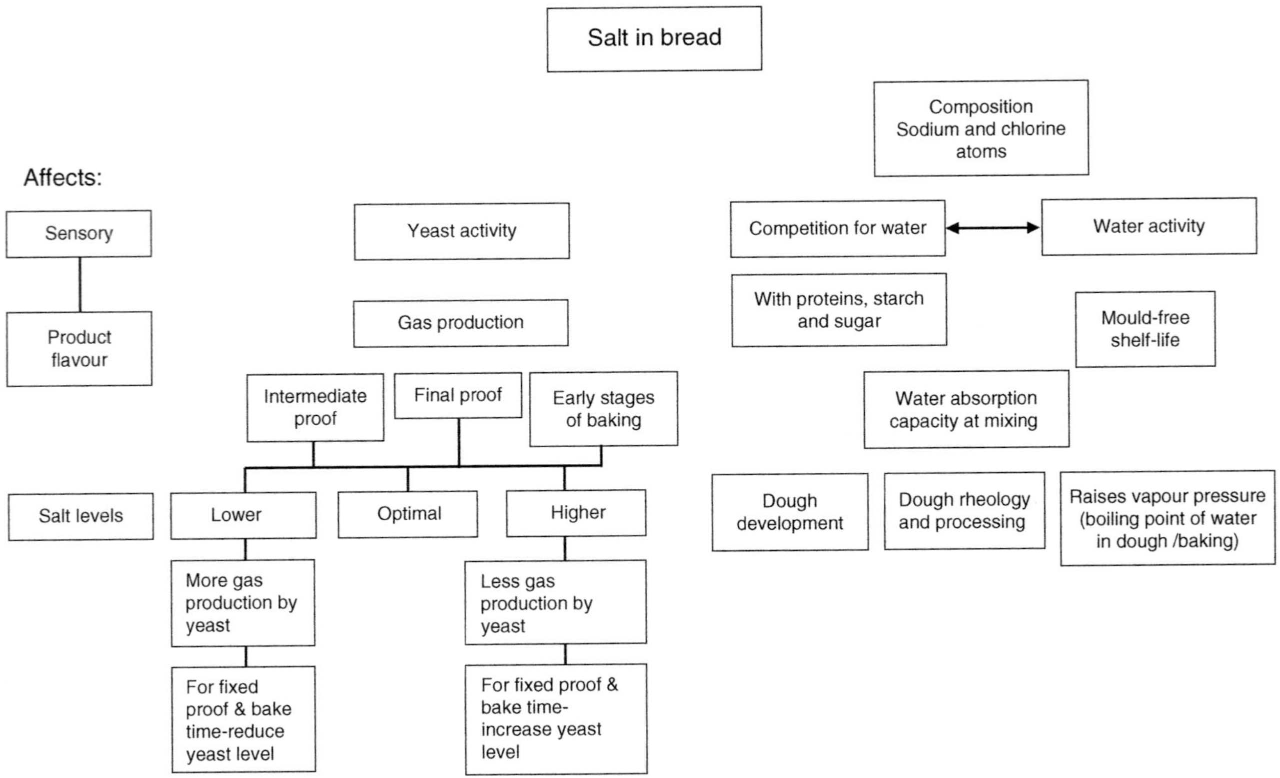

Figure 7.5 Knowledge fragment for salt in bread

suitable taste panels. Again, the reader is referred elsewhere for a discussion of suitable sensory panel assessment techniques (e.g. Kilcast 2004). Given how important texture and eating quality are to consumer acceptance of any products and nutritionally enhanced bakery products in particular, assessment of these particular properties should be built into the early stages of product development programs. Trained sensory panel assessments tend to be a time-consuming and costly exercise, and there can be an inclination to minimise this type of work, or to delay it until the later stages of the development program. The latter is a risky practice if there are major negative responses from the assessment as this can unduly delay the introduction of new products.

While there are a range of objective texture analysis techniques available, they mostly fail to completely mimic the chewing patterns of humans and so cannot be taken as absolute indicators of consumer sensory acceptance of eating qualities. There have been many attempts to link sensory and objective measurement of texture with perhaps the best known example being Texture Profile Analysis (TPA). Developed in the 1960s, TPA was based on the classification food texture using seven properties determined with sensory panels evaluating a wide range of foods (Szczesniak 1963a). These seven properties were then related to objective methods of analysis (Szczesniak 1963b), with further developments as instrumentation for analysing food texture became more widespread and more sophisticated (Bourne 1978). The application of sensory evaluation and the objective measurements of food properties have developed significantly in the last 50 years, but the basic approach to link sensory and objective measurement of food texture remains valid and important today, not least for developing nutritionally enhanced bakery products which will win acceptance with consumers.

Aligning the objective measurement of bakery food texture with the key sensory properties of nutritionally enhanced bakery foods allows product development to proceed at a greater pace, reducing waste of time and resources, and is more likely to deliver consumer acceptable products in the long run. A particular strength of objective measures of texture is that one is able to quickly track directions of change with successive recipe and process trials which in turn, permits the development of valuable heuristic rules for the manipulation of baked product recipes and assessing the impact of processing methods. Cauvain and Young (2006) suggested how such qualitative heuristic rules for changes in product texture may be represented using simple diagrams. For example, to be able to identify if a laminated product is becoming less flaky or whether a cake is less soft for eating, is valuable in itself and being able to characterise the product change with an appropriate number has even greater value.

7.6 Examples of Linking Sensory and Objectively Measured Qualities with Bakery Products

Some examples as to how sensory and objective measured product texture qualities may be used in product development will illustrate the strength of the approach. Cauvain and Young (2008) discussed work carried out at the FMBRA, Chorleywood, UK, related to the crispness of pork meat pies in the UK. The pie concerned comprised a savoury shortcrust pastry enclosing a pork meat filling. The consumer preference for the pie pastry was that it should be crisp eating and retain that crispness for several days after baking. Moisture migration from the meat filling to the pastry during storage is largely responsible for loss of crispness of the pastry casing. The portions of the pastry casing which suffer most from softening (loss of crispness) are the lid and the sidewalls. Migration of fat to the base limits the potential for moisture migration to that area. The sensory component of the study discussed by Cauvain and Young (2008) used a five-point Hedonic scale because such scales are easily understood by untrained assessors with little instruction on sensory panels. The descriptors for portions of the pastry casing (sidewall and lid pastry only) ranged from totally unacceptable (0 = soft) to wholly acceptable (4 = crisp) with a panel score of 2 indicating that the pastry was neither unacceptable nor acceptable. This sensory 'neutral point' was then linked with an objective evaluation of pastry hardness using a puncture test with an Instron texture analyser. The resulting plots for the correlation of the pastry with the force required to puncture the pastry are illustrated in Figure 7.6 with the neutral values (nv) indicated for both sidewall and base pastries. Having determined the forces associated with the nv in sensory terms, it became possible to determine many of the factors likely to have a major impact on the consumer acceptability of the pastry without the constant need for using consumer panels. In the context of improving the nutritional value of bakery products, the investigations were able to investigate the importance of type of fat

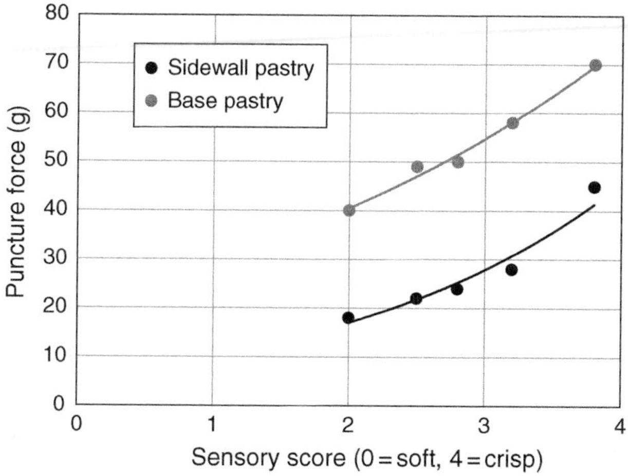

Figure 7.6 Relationship between sensory and objective data for pie pastry.

and its level in the preparation of the savoury shortcrust pastry shell, production methods, the impact of storage conditions and influence of wrapping materials.

A similar approach was used at FMBRA to study moisture migration in apple pies made with a sweetened short pastry. In this study additional information was gathered in that the moisture content of the pastry was measured at different moments in storage and an objective test was developed in which a narrow diameter blunt probe was driven downwards through the lid pastry, the pie filling and finally the base pastry in a continuous test. Cauvain (1992) illustrated the form of the test data that could be obtained. In this particular study the descriptors were chosen to study the panel perception of quality covering the degree to which the particular pastry component was liked or not. Thus, the scale ran from 1 (dislike a lot) to 5 (like a lot) with the neutral point being 3 (neither like nor dislike). A simple plot of mean panel ratings and mean pastry moisture content suggested that the neutral score was reached when the moisture content of the pastry was approximately 17%, and along with the relevant puncture data it was possible to identify the relative targets for puncture test data by which the study the impacts of ingredients and processing. As with the FMBRA studies of pork pies, moisture migration was again identified as the key process by which the shortcrust pastry softened. Unlike the savoury pie pastry discussed above, the presence of sugar in both the pastry and the apple filling offered a route for controlling the key driving force in moisture migration, namely the water activity of the components. Included in this study on apple pies were measures to reduce moisture migration, such as using barriers between the filling and the pastry (Cauvain 1995). In the context of seeking sugar reductions in bakery pastry products, this study emphasises the need for an holistic approach to recipe reformulation.

More recently Cauvain (*pers comm*) has been using a similar approach to investigate the commercial opportunities for the manufacture of reduced-fat doughnuts. In the case of doughnuts there are two sources of fat in the final products, that added in the dough formulation and that absorbed in the later stages of frying (Cauvain 2017a). The fat from both sources contributes to product volume, flavour, softness and shelf-life, so the acceptability constraints related to fat reduction are complex. The aim of the study was to evaluate if a reduction of overall fat content of the doughnut had an effect on the sensory properties of the final product, especially the perception of 'softness', which was known to be a key component in the consumer assessment of shelf-life in market places and the potential acceptability of a reduced fat doughnut by consumers. For the study a 5-point scale was used with descriptors ranging from 1 (very acceptable) to 5 (unacceptable); with 4 being slightly acceptable and being considered as the point at which the doughnut had reached the limit of its consumer shelf-life. The average acceptability scores for the trials are given in Table 7.3 and illustrated in Figure 7.7. The data show that the limit of consumer acceptability for this product was reached on day 4 after production. At the same time as sensory assessments were being carried out, the texture of samples of doughnuts were being tested out using a single compression technique with a texture analyser. The

Table 7.3 Average sensory scores for doughnut acceptability.

Day after production	Score
1	1
2	2.83
3	3.17
4	3.92
5	4.08

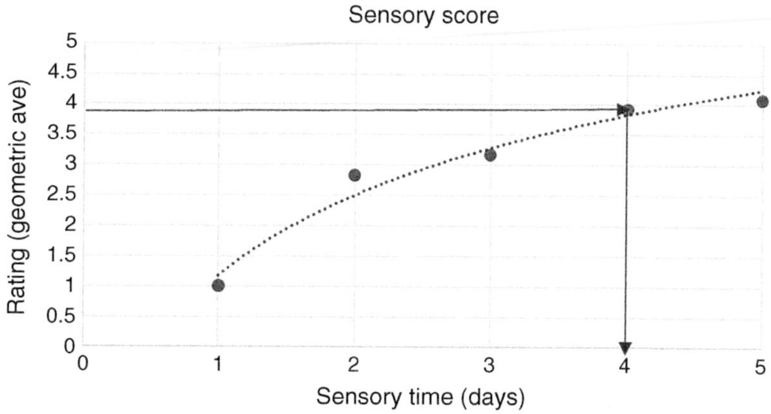

Figure 7.7 Average acceptability score of doughnuts with time after production.

objective texture analysis method was chosen based on a survey of consumers who indicated that doughnut 'softness' was the property that they most associated with product freshness (an assessment that is also commonly made with bread and cake crumb). The relationship between the sensory acceptability ratings and the objective texture data is illustrated in Figure 7.8 and it shows that for the standard doughnut formulation the compression area was approximately 1700 g.s. Using this figure as the objective limiting value for consumer acceptability, is was possible to limit the number of sensory trials required and carry out many variations in doughnut recipe and production methods in order to evaluate the most promising route for fat reduction. Though it did prove technically possible to make significant reductions in overall fat level in the doughnuts, it appeared from the objective data that the acceptability limit for the reduced-fat doughnut would be three days instead four. When samples of these lower fat level doughnuts were submitted for sensory testing, the panel confirmed that three days was the most likely limit of acceptability for the new product. While this was most certainly feasible technically, the manufacturer was faced with a practical problem in that a reduction of one day in sensory shelf-life had a negative impact on production scheduling due to the extended nature of the local distribution system. The unintended consequences of developing a 'healthier' doughnut in this example necessitated significant production changes in the bakery.

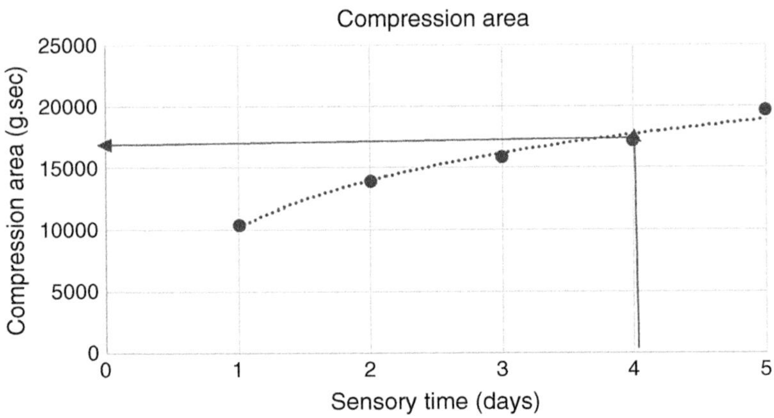

Figure 7.8 Relationship between sensory and objective data for doughnuts.

7.7 Strategies for Developing Product and Process Developments to Deliver Enhanced Nutrition

The development of practical strategies for delivering enhanced nutrition via bakery products inevitably starts with a clear identification as to what specific nutritional benefits are to be delivered by the final product, combined with a clear understanding of the market in which the products are to be placed. There is an understandable inclination in product development to start with an idea of incorporating 'healthy' ingredients into an existing range of products. This development approach faces a number of specific problems. The first is being able to deliver an identifiable nutritional benefit which can be substantiated in a bakery product. While there are some clearly identifiable ingredient-related health benefits, they may not always be deliverable at the end of the baking process following the long exposure of many ingredients to the harshness of baking oven conditions. The loss of water and the high temperatures to which product surfaces are exposed can lead to the breakdown of heat-sensitive nutritional components and perhaps the development of unwanted anti-health or anti-nutritional components (as discussed above). In the latter context the formation of acrylamide in carbohydrate-rich foods with the presence of the amino acid asparagine in the matrix, illustrates the potential at least, for unintended consequences in well-intended product developments.

Most food regulatory bodies around the world have some formal guidance or legislation related to the form and nature of health claims which are applicable and permissible to bakery foods. Many are already clearly stated and readily followed by food manufactures. Other claims may require approval in one form or another by relevant bodies (e.g. European Food Safety Authority), even necessitating considerable research work to identify and justify the basis of the claim. The nature of many health-related claims may be ascertained through a knowledge of a specific ingredient, for example, the potential for oat products to deliver cholesterol-lowering benefits because they are rich in *beta*-glucan, is well-established. The fact that such health claims may already exist establishes no certainty that they can be transferred without due consideration from one type of food to another. Clearly there will be some link between the claimed (established) benefit and the quantity consumed, usually on a daily basis. It may be the case that the incorporation of a particular 'healthy' ingredient from one food type to another is simply not possible because the levels required for typical servings may be impractical at best, or in many cases will negatively affect the desirable qualities of a product.

In terms of increasing the overall healthiness of bakery products, we have already seen that in many cases there is a reformulation conundrum which in practice, means that there are rarely single, 'magic' replacement ingredients. The product development process most commonly requires a 'systems solution' in which complex reformulations are often combined with alternative or new, processing methods. Claims related to the major nutritional inputs from bakery products (e.g. fat, saturated fat, sugar, fibre) are detailed for most if not all, parts of the world. There will also be clearly stated targets and definitions for low or reduced nutrients. The detail as to how such claims can be made may vary, but the limits which apply to the various claims will be clearly stated. The identification of such targets in the context new product development are an essential first step.

The initial brief for a new product should encompass all of the physical, chemical, nutritional and texture attributes which are relevant, along with the requirements for both sensory and microbial shelf-lives. This can represent a long list of requirements, as shown by the example in Table 7.4, which includes comments as to how the properties identified might be assessed. As far as possible, the emphasis with

Table 7.4 Example specification for a new bakery product.

Product property	Means of assessment
Dimensions (width, length, height)	Objective
Volume	Objective
Crust colour	Subjective and/or objective (e.g. tristimulus)
Crumb colour	Subjective and/or objective (e.g. tristimulus)
Crust hardness (if important)	Subjective and/or objective (texture analysis)
Crumb softness (if important)	Subjective and/or objective (texture analysis)
Crispness (if important)	Subjective and/or objective (texture analysis)
Flakiness (if important)	Subjective and/or objective (texture analysis)
Crumb structure (if important)	Subjective scoring and/or image analysis (e.g. C-Cell).
Moisture content	Objective analysis
Water activity	Objective analysis
Shelf-life – staling	Sensory, objective (texture analysis)
Shelf-life – microbial	Objective analysis
Nutritional profile	Objective analysis

product assessment should be by objective means. The product attribute list should be as complete as possible before any practical work is undertaken, to make the product development as efficient as possible. There are many other steps along the product development route which will have to be satisfied before product launch, but a comprehensive and clearly stated product descriptor at the start of the development is essential. As the nutritional attributes are to be an essential feature of the new product, the assembly of relevant nutritional data for the ingredients is a necessary first step. The assembled data should be compatible with the nutritional aims of the project. It is not always the case that ingredient suppliers readily supply the necessary data and it may be that supplementary information is required in order to complete this task. This may require involvement of the primary producer of a raw material rather than relying on a supplier, or often incomplete specification sheets. The primary producer involvement will certainly be necessary when it comes to some of the technologically functional properties of the raw materials. For example, while an ingredient specification for a source of fat may well indicate the proportion of saturated fat in the raw material, the solid fat profile (solid fat index or solid fat content) will have greater relevance with respect to the creaming properties of the material and its contribution to lift in the manufacture of laminated products (Cauvain 2017a).

7.8 Finding a 'Starting Point'

Since most bakery products have a long history of manufacture and associated consumer expectations, the starting point for developments is usually readily defined in broad terms; for example, a cup cake. This means that a starting recipe will be available for the standard product and it will be relatively easy to establish the existing nutritional profile of that product, if it is not already available. Nutritional profiles are a common requirement for packaged bakery products around the world and will include the proportions of each of the major food groups; fats with the proportion of saturated fats indicated separately, carbohydrates with the proportion of sugars indicated separately, protein and fibre. Sodium and salt equivalents are commonly stated. There will be variations on the stated nutritional profile according to local requirements and preferences. Energy values are commonly stated on a 'per 100 g', and 'per portion' basis, with the mass associated with the portion also being stated.

Having previously identified the nutritional targets for the new product it is a relatively easy step to identify the direction and magnitude of the nutritional changes in a 'standard' product required to deliver the new target. Once quantified, delivery of the nutritional targets needs to be viewed in relation to the list of available (permitted) ingredients. It is helpful to assemble a database of ingredients populated with data in the same format as will be used to define the nutritional values of final product; this makes the calculation of theoretical values straightforward and allows many recipe iterations to be carried out on the computer using appropriate calculation models. However, since the functionality of the ingredients is not taken into account, any product recipe defined solely by its nutritional composition is not guaranteed to succeed without further refinement.

One area constantly overlooked is that of ingredient and therefore recipe and product moisture content. Ingredient specifications sometimes do not state the ingredient moisture content. If this data is missing, then it may be possible to derive an approximate value by simply summing the mass of the other ingredients and assuming that the value required to make the total equal to 100 is derived from water. However, this simple approach is only appropriate if the ingredient specification is quoted on an 'as-is' basis and not a dry matter basis, as has been observed in a significant number of cases by the authors. As has already been discussed, water plays a major role in the creation of baked product matrices (dough, batter) and it as major contributor to product texture and shelf-life, both sensory and microbially-free (Cauvain and Young 2008). The final product moisture level is also important when it come to the energy values defined for the product, not least since water has no energy value. This zero-energy value has to be factored into the product energy calculations.

The important role that water plays in delivering the final product should be well appreciated, but the contribution of one important manufacturing step is often overlooked in product development (and indeed in bakery product manufacturing in general), namely the baking loss. All bakery products lose water as a result of baking and a knowledge of the baking loss is important for understanding product shelf-life. The baking loss for each bakery product should be measured for each set of baking conditions used and recorded. These values become useful when new recipe development iterations are carried out, as they are needed to deliver the most relevant nutritional data from recipe calculations. Baking losses can usually be calculated by simply weighing products before and after baking because water will be the major recipe component which has changed.

If a suitable tool or service is available, then it is possible to carry through each of the nutritionally modified recipes for an assessment of product water activity and an indication of mould-free shelf-life without making the product. In the case that a failure to reach the required mould-free shelf-life is indicated, then further manipulation of ingredients to deliver the relevant shelf-life can be carried out and then cross-checked with the nutritional calculations. While this may seem like a tedious and time-consuming activity, it is significantly faster than making products with every potential recipe change and measuring their water activities, or waiting for the product to go mouldy when stored under defined temperature conditions. Over the years much of the development of bakery products has relied on the 'trial and error' approach linked with product assessment carried out by relevant products experts. Indeed, this approach probably remains the most common method of new product development. Trial and error is time consuming and relies heavily on the skills of bakery experts. If the time and resources are available, then the trial and error approach is a good way to assemble a range of product development skills. Time tends to be a limited resource in the product development world and this may contribute to the apparent lack of progress in developing healthier bakery products. Once a promising products recipe has been identified, it may be appropriate to undertake a test bake in order to make an early evaluation of the likely product outcome and to cross-check calculated and measured analytical data.

While the nutritional profile and to some extent, the microbial shelf-life of a product can be based on calculated or modelled data, the same is not true to any significant extent for the 'functional' properties of ingredients, their interactions in recipes and potential impacts of processing dimension in the manufacture of bakery products. The 'tools' available for modelling such important issues tend to be limited in nature and this area of activity remains very much the province of the 'expert'. Some of the potential visualisation tools have been identified above and a product development expert may well establish their own library of such information, actual or virtual, populated with the necessary heuristic rules on which to base a development program. However, the introduction of less well known raw materials in functionality terms, may significantly challenge the established heuristic models and test baking remains a necessary and important way in which to systematically gather the data within new product development.

Cauvain and Young (2006, 2008) suggested techniques which can aid the product development process, and these were revised by Cauvain (2017b). It is relevant to note that reformulation of recipes to meet nutritional recommendations may require the implementation of changes to existing process technologies, or the development of alternative ones in order to deliver a final product of a quality which will be accepted by consumers. The introduction of a processing dimension to the reformulation conundrum adds significantly to the challenges involved in product development and the implementation of recipe changes in a commercial environment. The latter consideration is especially important since most industrial bakery plants lack flexibility of manufacture and the extension or modification of existing plants is not a trivial exercise. Thus, while a successful formulation may be achieved, it may prove impossible to manufacture the product concerned. This restriction almost certainly limits opportunities for the development of some healthier bakery products, or at least slows down the commercialisation processes involved. The early identification of relevant processing issues and options requires a comprehensive understanding of relevant bakery processing technology. As far as possible, processing requirements and options should be incorporated into the initial product brief, not least so that any potential capital equipment requirements are identified early in the product development process.

7.9 Continuing the Development Process

Many bakery products are defined by a mixture of apparently conflicting properties which commonly means that relatively small changes in the choice of an ingredient, or its level in a recipe, can result in major shifts in product quality. The complex interactions which characterise the manufacture of bakery products become more so when a nutritional dimension is added to product specifications. For example, if a low salt level is specified for the final product, it is necessary to consider all sources of sodium in the recipe in order to identify the magnitude of the change required for recipe salt. In some product developments, particularly those where chemical aeration is a key process requirement (e.g. biscuits, cakes), the requirement for low salt in the final product may lead to elimination of sodium chloride from the recipe altogether, with potential negative effects on taste and microbial shelf-life. Other ingredient and recipe changes may have more far-reaching impacts than this 'relatively' simple example of salt reduction. For example, the replacement of a high melting point fat with an oil has a negative impact on dough gas retention in breadmaking (leading to low volume), will reduce the air incorporation in cake batters potentially necessitating the use of an emulsifier (such as glycerol monostearate), and prevent the formation of a laminated structure in puff pastry.

As the development of a new product continues, test baking will deliver significant quantities of process and product data which have direct value for identifying relevant next steps. There are many well-known and appropriate statistical processes which may be applied to the development process, some of which have been commented on above. However, there is a difference between establishing a study to determine statistically significant effects in baking and the practical needs for product development, with the latter often requiring a more pragmatic approach to data analysis, not least because of the inevitable time pressures. A statistical study can provide much of the background data required for the significant effects of ingredients and bakery processes, but often new product development is associated with effects that may lack 'statistical significance', yet are significant in the delivery of the required end-product. This is not to suggest that quantification of data from test bakes is not important, quite the reverse, rather to say that more critical in product development is the ability to understand whether a change has been introduced and whether that change is consistent with the product targets or not, or whether it has introduced other unintended product quality effects, positive or negative.

Watching for and identifying patterns in data during product development are helpful in achieving the relevant product targets. There are a number of techniques which may be applied, one of which is through the use of 'spider' diagrams, a technique often associated with sensory analysis, but which can be readily populated with any number of product attributes. An example of such a diagram is illustrated in Figure 7.9 in which a standard and reduced-fat cake are compared. A set of critical 'target' properties have been identified and linked to form the diagram. Test baking data associated with the new product development concerned have been introduced and so it is possible to see to what extent the new product pattern matches or deviates from

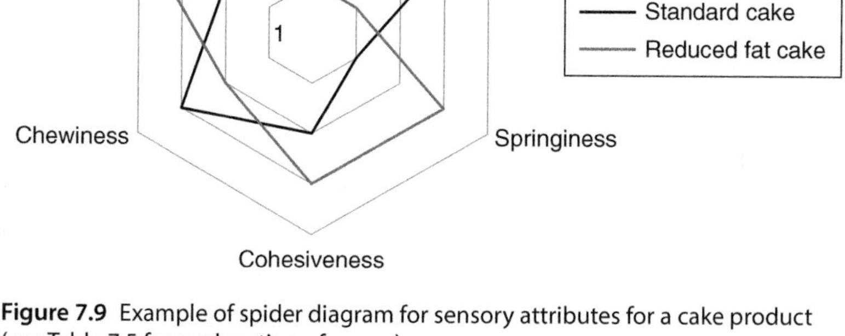

Figure 7.9 Example of spider diagram for sensory attributes for a cake product (see Table 7.5 for explanation of scores).

Table 7.5 Sensory scoring attributes for cakes illustrated in Figure 7.9.

Cake sensory property	Score of 1	Score of 5
Fracturability	Difficult to break apart	Breaks apart very easily
Firmness	Very firm	Very soft
Springiness	Springs back readily	Does not spring back
Cohesiveness	Does not crumble in mouth	Crumbles in mouth
Chewiness	Very chewy	Not chewy
Gumminess	Very gummy	Not gummy

the target. Adjustment of the recipe for a subsequent test bake will most likely still require the intervention of a human expert (at least for the immediate future in the baking industry), but subsequent test bakes will continue to contribute to the development of a rule base on which the final new product and process specification can be based.

If data have been gathered from multiple test bakes but no exact match with the target values for the new product has been achieved, support for identifying the basis for further test baking may be obtained by assessing the closeness of existing results with the proposed target. Clustering analysis is one supporting technique that may be applied. A common approach is to construct a dendogram using product attribute data to indicate which test variation(s) is closest to the target and so might form the basis for further developments. An example of a dendogram being used in product development is illustrated in Figure 7.10. In this example the impact of a mixed enzyme formulation is being assessed against a defined combination of dough rheology and bread characteristics for a series of wheat flours. While this example is not directly focussed on the development of a nutritionally enhanced bakery product it does illustrate another means for handling multiple data points in the development process.

7.10 Identifying Processing Options

Less easily identified in the development of nutritionally enhanced bakery products are changes to the manufacturing processes which may have beneficial impacts related to the delivery of the final product.

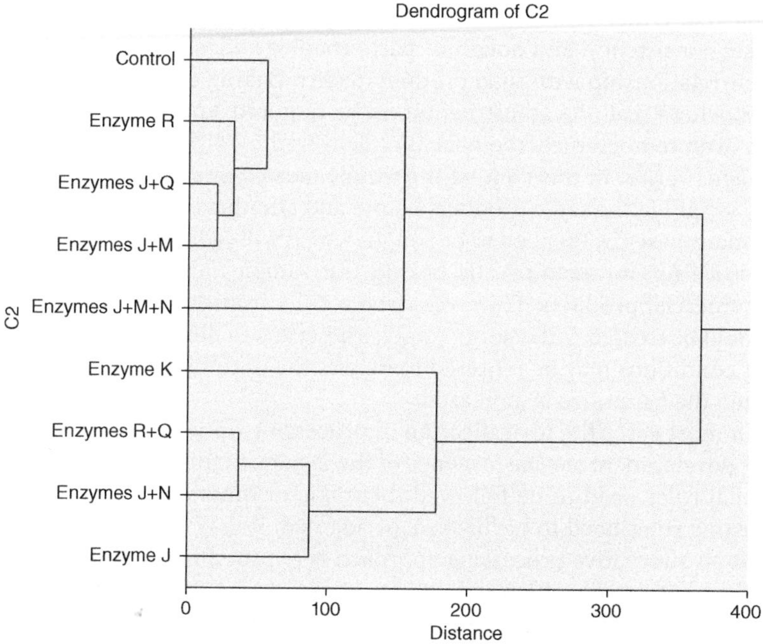

Figure 7.10 Example of a dendogram used in the evaluation of enzyme–flour interactions in breadmaking.

Processing models for bakery products are less well studied, defined or developed than formulation options for existing, standard bakery products, let alone for new developments. As noted above, the potential means by which the product may be manufactured at the end of the development process should be included in the initial project brief, so that the move to commercial production is not unduly delayed with processing problems. The 'scale-up' of a product from kitchen or test bakery, to manufacturing plant is often one of the most difficult stages in all new product development because the recipe-process interactions are quite different at the different scales, even if the equipment used is of the same nominal design.

At the early stages of the development cycle, it is important to gather data which may be used for process control at the manufacturing stage, and to identify the technical critical control points. Common examples of critical points include batter density to assess the level of aeration which is desirable and achieved, so that mixing times may be adjusted. Other critical measurements may include dough, batter or paste consistency, and dough or paste rheology, ideally together with their relationship with final product quality. Baking conditions is one area where scale-up adjustments will be required since for a nominal set oven temperature, the heat flux delivered by different ovens and designs varies. In this context the simple measurement of weight loss (by weighing the same products before and after baking) is invaluable. In many cases, ways need to be sought which will reduce the problems of scale-up; for example, by baking test samples alongside existing commercial products. However, even results from such an approach should be treated with caution, not least because a different set of baking conditions may be required to deliver the optimised new product when the batch size is increased.

In most cases the identification of processing options in new product development are the province of the expert, in this case to identify which rules need to be followed (heuristic or otherwise), and which existing rules need to be 'broken' or adapted. It may even be the case that an alternative processing approach is required in order to establish a platform on which to build a successful new and healthier bakery product. There are no guidelines which can be quoted for approaching the development of novel processing methods in baking, we are now considering an area where humans operate more effectively than modelling or mathematical techniques. This is truly the area of 'Let's try it and see what happens', a place where every result is important in developing an improved knowledge-base. However, the successful development of a new processing method on the kitchen scale still faces the hurdles associated with scale-up to commercial scale, particularly so if the equipment required for the new processing method is not immediately available. In each new product brief, some room should be left to allow adaptions or innovative processing options as they may be the option which ultimately delivers a successful development.

7.11 Verifying Nutritional Targets

It is a statement of the obvious that if healthier bakery products are to be developed, then there must be a means of verifying that the products meet any identified nutritional targets when sold. Analytical techniques are well-established, with agreed international standard methods covering all of the requirements that would be associated with nutritionally enhanced bakery products. While the recipe development process may be based on theoretical calculations, it is important that relevant measurements are made periodically throughout the product development, if only to avoid being faced with a major discrepancy at the point of manufacture. Despite the analytical techniques being well-established, the verification of nutritional data is not without its challenges, which include:

- *Choice of samples*
  Few bakeries will produce products which are 100% identical; potential variations are associated with both batch-to-batch and within batch variability. There can also be a within-day variability (often from drift or shift changes) and day-to-day changes. Steps should be taken to ensure that samples chosen for analytical testing are representative of the 'typical' production. The variability of sample weight in production should be known so that the risks associated with any claims which involve portion size can be identified; e.g. the energy delivered per portion. Variations in product moisture content which typically arise from baking should be known and factored into the choice of samples for testing.
- *Sample preparation and sub-sampling*
  The majority of bakery products have a degree of heterogeneity in their structure. At the macro-level this can be associated with the inclusions such as pieces of fruits or nuts, and at the micro-level this can be associated with moisture gradients in the baked product (lower crust and higher crumb moisture). In all cases before measuring the analytical composition, a product must be reduced to a suitable form for subsequent sub-sampling, with care being taken that the preparation of the material does not affect its analytical composition (commonly loss or gain of moisture).
- *Sources of error*
  Assuming that the preparation of the sample has been adequately carried out, then it should be the case that any sub-samples which are taken from the bulk sample are representative of the whole. However, no analytical method is without its sources of error. This means that even if the sub-samples were identical in composition, there could still be apparent differences in composition between replicate sub-samples. For approved standard methods such measurement errors will be known and identified, and should be quoted with all analytical measurements.

- *Assumptions with energy calculations*
  Food energy values are not normally measured but calculated from the compositional data, using agreed energy values for carbohydrates, protein and fat. However, it should be recognised that such calculations are commonly based on values derived from analytical data which, as noted above, are subject to measurement errors. The risks associated with variations in sample weight and moisture content have also been noted above and need to factored into claims related to product energy values. It should also be noted that some ingredients which may potentially be used in the manufacture of healthier baker products, will have different energy values than those commonly used in nutritional calculations (typically lower); such differences will need to be taken into account when calculating energy values.

7.12 Conclusions

The development of nutritionally enhanced bakery products requires a range of inputs in order to deliver a potentially successful product in a commercial environment. Whatever the development approaches deployed, a key first step will be a clear definition as to what the nutritional 'targets' are for the proposed products, combined with other attributes including the physical appearance, specific textural attributes and shelf-life requirements. Alternatives to the classical 'trial-and-error' approach in product development should be sought at the beginning of the development process. The potential for employing both quantitative and qualitative models should be explored; most likely a combination of the two modelling approaches will aid the development approach. At any early stage the potential contribution of processing options should be examined with sufficient thought being given to the potential for beneficial changes to existing processing methods. It will be important to quickly establish the need to adapt existing processing equipment, or seek the development of new technologies. A likely consequence of the modification of existing product formulations, especially those which involve a reduction or replacement of key functional ingredients such as fat and sugar, is that the new products becomes more 'process-sensitive'. Verification of the progress towards achieving the proposed nutrition targets should be sought throughout the development process.

References

BakeTran (2012) A guide to the effects of the main ingredients used cake and sponge recipes. *Chorleywood Bookshelf Monograph No. 3*, www.baketran.com/

Bent, A.J. (1997). *The Technology of Cake Making*, 6e. London, UK: Blackie Academic & Professional.

Bourne, M.C. (1978). Texture profile analysis. *Food Technology* 32: 62–66, 72.

Cauvain, S.P. (1992). Evaluating the texture of baked products. *South African Bakery and Confectionary Review* 30: 20–28.

Cauvain, S.P. (1995). Putting pastry under the microscope. *Baking Industry Europe* 68–69.

Cauvain, S.P. (2015). *Technology of Breadmaking*, 3e. Switzerland: Springer International Publishing.

Cauvain, S.P. (2017a). *Baking Problems Solved*, 2e. Duxford, UK: Woodhead Publishing.

Cauvain, S.P. (2017b). *The ICC Handbook of Cereals, Flour, Dough and Product Testing: Methods and Applications*. Lancaster, PA: DES*tech* Publications.

Cauvain, S.P. and Young, L.S. (2006). *Baked Products: Science, Technology and Practice*. Oxford, UK: Blackwell Publishing.

Cauvain, S.P. and Young, L.S. (2008). *Bakery Food Manufacture and Quality: Water Control and Effects*, 2e. Oxford, UK: Wiley-Blackwell.

Kilcast, D. (2004). *Texture in Food; Volume 1 Consumers, Texture and Food Quality*. Cambridge, UK: Woodhead Publishing.

Meilgaard, M.C., Civille, G.V., and Carr, B.T. (2016). *Sensory Evaluation Techniques*, 5e. New York, NY: Taylor & Francis Group, LLC.

Street, C.A. (1991). *Flour Confectionery Manufacture*. Glasgow, UK:: Blackie.

Szczesniak, A.S. (1963a). Classification of textural characteristics. *Journal of Food Science* 28: 385–389.

Szczesniak, A.S. (1963b). Objective measurement of food texture. *Journal of Food Science* 28: 410–420.

Thomas Hedley & Co. Ltd (1958). *Formula Rebalance*, 3e. Manchester, UK: Thomas Hedley & Co. Ltd Research Department.

Young, L.S. (1995). Getting the product right. *Food Manufacture* 43.

Young, L.S. (1996). Developing flour confectionery products. *The European Food and Drink Review* 41–44.

Young, L.S. (2007). Application of baking knowledge in software systems. In: *Technology of Breadmaking*, 2e (ed. S.P. Cauvain and L.S. Young), 207–222. New York, NY: Springer Science+Business Media, LLC.

Young, L.S., Davies, P.R., and Cauvain, S.P. (1998). Cakes – getting the right balance. In: *Applications and Innovations in Expert Systems VI* In: Proceedings of the 18th Annual Conference of the British Computer Society Specialist Group on Expert Systems, Cambridge, December 1998. (ed. A. Mackintosh), 42–55. Cambridge, UK: SGES Publications.

8

Communicating Relevant Messages

8.1 Introduction

As has been noted several times above, the development of nutritionally enhanced bakery products is no guarantee of their acceptance in the marketplace. Much of the previous discussion has focussed on the need to understand consumer requirements for such products and the ability of the baking industry to deliver them with the required sensory properties in order to gain consumer acceptance. This combination of understanding and ability to deliver is essential if relevant health and dietary benefits are to be passed on to consumers. In the context of the development of nutritionally enhanced products, it is important to recognise that a key element in gaining product acceptance is through conveying relevant and accurate messages regarding the products and their associated health benefits. Such information has to be in a form which can be readily understood and assimilated by consumers. This is not a simple task, not least because of the diversity of consumers and the wide range of potential communication methods which might be used. Equally there needs to be a common understanding between health professionals and bakery food manufacturers so that the messages are clear and unequivocal; for many reasons this has not always been the case. Nutrition and food-health related studies are important for improving the well-being of humankind (Carlisle and Hanlon 2014). However, the results of many of these studies may be equivocal and these raise uncertainties in the minds of food manufacturers as to the validity and relevance of the information which they receive and how they should act on it in the development

Baking Technology and Nutrition: Towards a Healthier World, First Edition.
Stanley P. Cauvain and Rosie H. Clark.

of nutritionally enhanced products. The understanding and application of nutrition and health-studies are not helped by the manner in which they are sometimes communicated through the media and marketing, as noted in a critical analysis presented by Jackson et al. (2014). Communications from special interest groups may not always be clear which can lead to longer-term misunderstandings with consumers (Cauvain 2003). Such situations further compound uncertainties in the food industry as to which nutritional objectives should be addressed, how they should be delivered and crucially, how they might be communicated to potential consumers.

The lack of clarity as to what constitutes a 'healthy' food is compounded by what constitutes an 'unhealthy' food. Labels such as 'junk', 'convenience', and 'processed' foods were and still are, commonly used in the media to 'simplify' messages for consumers. While this might be expected from the popular media, such ad hoc labelling of food categories has also invaded the academic and pseudo-academic communities. Clearly all foods have some health benefits, not least since the lack of food is most certainly unhealthy. Equally clear is that some foods, including those popularly classified as manufactured or processed foods, have greater health benefits than others. Almost no food has the complete and perfect nutrition for consumers and so the consensus view amongst health professionals over a long period of time, has been and remains, that an individual diet should comprise a mixture of food sources to deliver the required nutrition. Implicit is the recognition that the structure of that diet may vary as individuals pass through the various stages in their life (Hegarty 1992). With the correct focus on the healthiness of the diet, it is easier to understand the contribution that individual foods can make to the healthy diet.

Access to basic data relevant to diet and health has increased dramatically in the last couple of decades or so, not least because of the advent of the internet and other modern means of mass communication. This increased access to information for all is not without its risks; at best it can lead to some uncertainty as to what information is relevant, and at its worst it can lead to the dissemination of information that is simply 'wrong'. Accessing relevant data is only the first step in developing an understanding of diet and health, the next and more critical step, is placing it into its relevant contexts. Put simply, the interpretation of the information and the data which are presented are probably more important than accessing it. With the plethora of information available on diet and health, there is a danger of us all becoming 'experts' on the subject. Equally, as discussed above, our knowledge regarding diet and health continues to evolve so that we can anticipate even more information on the subject being made available as time moves on. Accessing more information does not improve its relevance and often in doing so highlights the uncertainties and contradictions of individual pieces of nutritionally related information.

8.2 Communicating Nutrition and Health Information on Relevant Food Sources

Basic dietary information on what constitutes a healthy diet is largely the responsibility of government-led initiatives and actions around the world. While the various initiatives and actions may be implemented at a local level, they are commonly linked with major initiatives within organisations like the World Health Organization (WHO). The WHO brings together health and nutrition experts to tackle dietary and health problems, and create improved awareness on a global scale. While many will be aware of WHO initiatives in tackling malnutrition, they may be less aware of their contributions to those common global problems related to excess or inappropriate energy intakes. The position of the WHO on global issues related to the current challenges of increasing obesity in many populations has been referred to above.

Communicating basic dietary information to consumers is most commonly carried out at a local geographical level, so that the messages can focus on the most relevant food sources and dietary requirements for different populations in different locations. Often the basic information is communicated using diagrams in which food sources are ranked or visually displayed according to their contributions to the local diet and suggested frequency of consumption. A common form is the 'food' pyramid. In a pyramid guide, the more important foods in human nutrition and health form the base, indicating their significant importance in delivering the required nutrition and the potentially high frequency of their consumption. The further up the pyramid that a food source is, the lower the recommended frequency of consumption. Often the positioning of the food source on the food pyramid is related to its composition and contribution to total energy value, with foods higher up the pyramid contributing less valued nutrition (e.g. higher in fat and sugar, lower in fibre). Bakery products which are significant contributors to a healthy diet, such as wholemeal bread because of its positive contribution to fibre in the diet, may be seen at the pyramid base while those which contain higher levels of fat and sugar (e.g. biscuits, cakes, pastries) will occur at a higher level. An alternative to the pyramid is the 'pie' chart, an example of which is published in the UK as the Eatwell guide (www.gov.uk/government/publications/the-eatwell-guide). In this case the sizes of the pie slices relate to the nutritional value in the diet and frequency of consumption. Further advice is given as to the type of the food to eat sparingly, for bakery products this includes biscuits, cookies and cakes. Food pyramids and similar dietary information devices may be linked with more focussed advice on a specific area of nutrition. An example promoted by the National Health Service (NHS) in the UK has been the '5 a day' message which was designed to encourage the consumption of five daily portions of dietary fibre delivered with simplified messages as to the relevant sources of dietary fibre (www.nhs.uk/live-well/eat-well/why-5-a-day). The advice given in the NHS program was based on WHO recommendations for eating a minimum of 400 g of fruit and vegetables a day to lower the risk of serious health problems, such as heart disease, stroke, and some cancers. The advice included the clarification that the five portions should be a mix of fruit and veg and not five portions of each.

When considering diet, health and nutrition it should be done within the context of the lifestyle of individuals. In its most basic form the relevant information is conveyed in terms of a 'typical' or 'recommended' daily energy intake, usually expressed as kilocalories (kcal) or kilojoules (kJ) per day. Recommended daily dietary energy intake levels vary slightly around the world but most stand around 2500 kcal for adult males and 2000 for adult females. The recommended levels will often be linked with lifestyle, with lower daily intakes being associated with and recommended for sedentary lifestyles, and higher levels for active ones. In essence the daily recommended intakes work on the principle that energy taken-in should not exceed energy used, so that a healthy adult neither gains nor loses weight throughout their lives. Recommendations for infants, children, and pregnant women will differ. There is a general consensus that, in many parts of the world, levels of activity associated with adult work have fallen progressively in recent years, so that less food and drink energy is required to maintain a healthy body mass balance. Recognition of this change has had an impact on our consideration of the recommended levels of daily energy intake, though advice on the subject has largely remained unchanged (in the UK at least) since the 1950s when lifestyles for most individuals were significantly different from those of the present day.

In addition to communicating basic nutrition and health messages, there may be a need to deliver specific advice to consumers on micronutrients (sometimes also referred to as 'trace elements' and minerals). Such guidance may be specific to a particular nutrient or aimed at specific sectors of populations; for example, in the latter case the provision of information on folic acid to pregnant women or those intending to become pregnant (www.bda.uk.com/foodfacts/FolicAcid.pdf). As with basic nutrition information, the guidance on micronutrients will come from official sources, such as the WHO or local government institutions. Commonly, relevant health and nutrition and health-related organisations publish summaries of their advice and guidance as pamphlets accessible on the web which include the background information on which the advice is based. Readers are referred elsewhere for a more detailed consideration of the role of micronutrients (Prasad 2011).

8.3 Communication of Basic Dietary Information by Food Manufacturers

The requirements placed upon food manufacturers to communicate dietary information to consumers is inevitably determined by local geographical requirements and legislation. Such requirements will most commonly specify the nature and form of the dietary information to be displayed, its location on the packaging and the format and font sizes to be used for the wording. For products which are for sale in more than one geographical location, multiple language versions may be required. In addition to the basic dietary information discussed in the context of this work, there will be requirements for the nature of ingredient descriptions and a declaration of allergens. Food labelling is a complex topic and outside the scope of this work; readers involved with labelling requirements should check with local legislative requirements and seek local guidance as appropriate. Increasingly there is a global commonality regarding the nature of the information displayed on the food pack but in the development of new products destined for more than one geographical market, care must be taken to ensure that all likely legislative requirements have been met.

Legislation with respect to food labelling is being constantly updated and should be checked carefully and early in the product development process, to avoid unnecessary waste of resources.

Consistent with an energy-based daily diet, the vast majority of packaged foods have an information panel on the pack which clearly states the energy value per 100 g of product. Energy values for portions or 'typical' servings may also be given (see example in Figure 6.3). The purpose of such information is to help consumers identify the contribution that a particular food and the quantity consumed will make to their total daily energy intake. Other means of communicating product energy information to consumers without making a particular nutrition claim, include front-of-pack energy content or serving (see example illustrated in Figure 8.1). Such approaches potentially increase consumer awareness of the contribution of portions of particular foods and products to their overall daily dietary intake. Claims related to reduced and low energy density foods and the means of communicating such information, are strictly regulated at a local geographical level (for example, in the EU see https://ec.

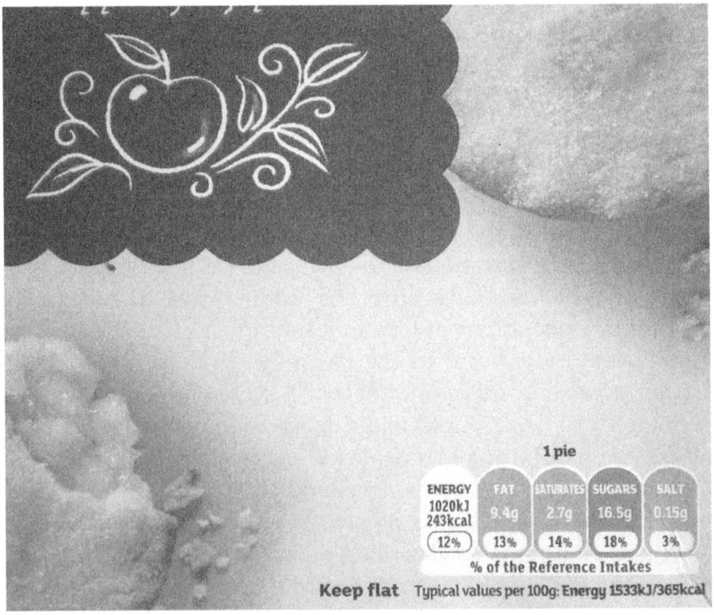
1 pie
ENERGY
1020kJ
243kcal
12%
FAT
9.4g
13%
SATURATES
2.7g
14%
SUGARS
16.5g
18%
SALT
0.15g
3%
% of the Reference Intakes
Keep flat
Typical values per 100g: Energy 1533kJ/365kcal

Figure 8.1 Example of 'front of pack' nutrition information.

europa.eu/food/safety/labelling_nutrition/claims/nutrition_claims_en). Possible claims related to the macronutrient composition of bakery products are further discussed below.

In addition to the total energy intake, it has become common practice to declare the composition of the product in terms of the major food components and the relevant nutritional values. An example of a common form for such a declaration is given in Table 8.1 for a cake product. These compositional data may be extended to include information related to a 'reference intake' (RI), or 'reference daily intake' (RDI) for an individual nutrient. An alternative to using RDIs is the 'traffic-light system' seen on some product packs in the UK and elsewhere. This is an attempt to produce more immediately recognisable nutritional information, with a 'green' flash indicating a nutrient that may be freely consumed, 'amber' less freely and 'red' occasionally. In many cases the traffic light scheme is carried on the front of the product pack to improve visibility and consumer awareness to make informed choices in the context of their diet and lifestyle. An example of the traffic light scheme is illustrated for a cake product in Figure 6.2. Examples of both approaches to conveying simplified front-of-pack nutritional information (traffic light and RDI) can be seen in the UK and elsewhere. In some cases, the traffic light scheme may relate the macronutrient composition of the product to the percentage of RI, as illustrated in Figure 8.2. The RDI information on product packs has,

Table 8.1 Example of a common form of ingredient declaration for a bakery product (Scrummmptious Cranberry and Orange Cake Bites, see Figure 4.3).

Typical values	Per 100 g	Per cake (30 g)
Energy	1310 kJ 311 kcal	390 kJ 93 kcal
Fat	12.2 g	3.7 g
of which saturates	4.4 g	1.3 g
Carbohydrates	36.0 g	11.0 g
of which sugars	19.1 g	5.7 g
Fibre	3.1 g	0.9 g
Protein	9.6 g	2.9 g
Salt	0.23 g	0.07 g

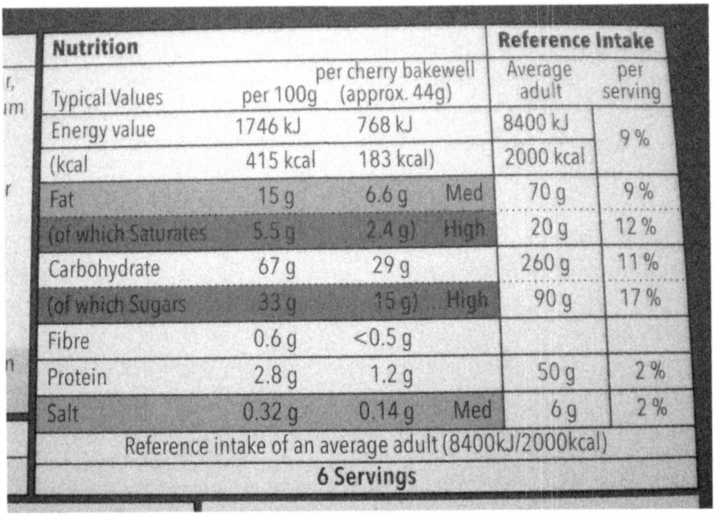

Nutrition				Reference Intake	
Typical Values	per 100g	per cherry bakewell (approx. 44g)		Average adult	per serving
Energy value	1746 kJ	768 kJ		8400 kJ	9%
(kcal	415 kcal	183 kcal)		2000 kcal	
Fat	15 g	6.6 g	Med	70 g	9%
(of which Saturates	5.5 g	2.4 g)	High	20 g	12%
Carbohydrate	67 g	29 g		260 g	11%
(of which Sugars	33 g	15 g)	High	90 g	17%
Fibre	0.6 g	<0.5 g			
Protein	2.8 g	1.2 g		50 g	2%
Salt	0.32 g	0.14 g	Med	6 g	2%
Reference intake of an average adult (8400kJ/2000kcal)					
6 Servings					

Figure 8.2 Macronutrient composition and reference intake information.

in many places, replaced the concept of Guideline Daily Amounts (GDA) introduced as a government-industry collaboration which began in 1998. In the USA Reference Daily Amounts (RDA) were used before moving to RDI. The change from GDA and RDA to RDI and the traffic light scheme, are all attempts to provide greater clarity of dietary information for consumers. The term Percentage Daily Value (%DV) may also be encountered in some (often older) literature, as may Daily Reference Intakes (DRI) and other acronyms related to dietary requirements; readers interested in obtaining a greater understanding of such nutritional terms are referred elsewhere (e.g. Devaney and Barr 2002).

8.4 Macronutrient Claims and Product Composition

In the development of nutritionally enhanced bakery products the ability to make particular health-related claims is important for the food producer. Health claims involving macronutrients may be linked with reductions in the levels of the major macronutrients fat, sugar and salt, increases in protein or fibre, or the use of specific forms of macronutrients, e.g. types of fats. Macronutrient claims will be the subject of specific regulation, the details of which will vary in different geographical areas and readers are advised to check local definitions and regulations. The decision to make a specific health-related claim and a check on local regulation should be performed at the start of the product development process, with regular checks being carried out to identify any potential changes which may affect the development process. While specific details related to claims may vary, a common theme of regulation will be that claims should not mislead consumers and be verifiable, often by independent means.

Commonly, claims for lower levels of macronutrients will be linked with terms such as 'reduced', 'low', 'very low', 'no added-', or '-free'. Bakery ingredients are most likely to fall into such categories are fat, sugar and salt. The levels by which such ingredients must fall to permit the use of the term 'reduced' will be defined in local legislation, with values of reduction being in the order of 25–30% or more, of the initial value. One of the commercial problems associated with the manufacture of a reduced version of a standard bakery product in order to convey 'healthiness', can be the registration in consumers' minds that the original version of the product was to some extent, unhealthy. Reduced ingredient versions of standard products may introduce greater variety into the product range, but it is not guaranteed that the introduction of a healthier version will result in increased sales, especially if consumers switch from one version to another. The maximum levels of macronutrients required to be present for products to classified as 'low' or 'very low' will be prescribed in most legislation based on weight per weight for solid foods, or weight per volume for liquids. There may be a limited variation for different foodstuffs; e.g. low fat in the EU is defined as 3 g per 100 g for solids, 1.5 g per 100 ml for liquids and 1.8 g per 100 ml of semi-skimmed milk.

Fat-, saturated fat-, sugar-, and salt-(sodium) free commonly have prescribed levels for solid and liquid foods. The position with respect to 'no added X' tends to be more complicated since many bakery ingredients may contain intrinsic levels of the specified macronutrient 'X'. Wheat flour is a good example of the issue since it contains low levels of intrinsic fat, sugars and sodium, so that while it could be possible to remove ingredient X from the product recipe, analytically X may be identified. Using the term 'no added sugar' will apply to any type of sugar, not just sucrose, if it is added as a separate ingredient and may need some qualification related to the occurrence of naturally occurring sugars which are part of another recipe ingredient.

Increases in macronutrient levels which have positive health connotations are most often those related to fibre, protein and specific fatty acids. They tend to be covered by terms such as 'high' or 'a source of' and will be covered by prescribed levels of the macronutrient concerned for both categories. The addition and use of *omega*-3 fatty acids, mono-unsaturated, poly-unsaturated, and unsaturated fats may permit health claims to be made; again the levels of use which will allow a claim to be made will be prescribed in local legislation.

Low energy and energy-free will have maximum prescribed levels for the energy value of the material or foodstuff. Claims for 'energy-reduced' will have to meet a prescribed reduction in energy density of a foodstuff; commonly this will be around a 30% reduction and may require a qualification of the characteristics which have allowed the energy reduction to be achieved. The terms 'light' and 'lite' are in common usage with a range of foods and drinks and are readily recognised by consumers around the world. Legislation related to the use of these terms is commonly (though not exclusively) benchmarked with the term 'reduced'. While in common usage for foodstuffs and drinks, it is not altogether clear as to whether consumers appreciate the specific nature of the energy reduction with common dictionary definitions referring to a product with 'fewer' calories.

8.5 Micronutrient Claims

Micronutrient claims are normally related to vitamins and minerals. In all cases claims related to specific micronutrients will refer to presence of a 'high' level of the specified substance which may occur 'naturally' as the result of the use of some ingredients, or through the deliberate addition of the specified substance in order to raise the level of named micronutrients. The descriptors allowed for micronutrient claims will inevitably be specified by local legislation. Some terms and definitions in common usage are:

- Source of micronutrient XX – typically the level of the specified micronutrient will need to meet a prescribed standard commonly identified as a 'significant amount'.
- High in micronutrient XX – the specified micronutrient will need to be present at prescribed higher level than for 'source of'. In many parts of the world a high level of a micronutrient would be taken as being twice the source of level.

- Contains micronutrient XX – typically this term is less well-defined, but a common legislative practice is to equate this term with 'source of' to avoid misleading consumers.
- Fortified with micronutrient XX – this term may be encountered under some legislative regimes when ingredients which have been used in the product have been fortified with specific micronutrients, e.g. flour. It may also be encountered where specific micronutrients have been deliberately added to the product formulation at levels which would be greater than might typically occur through the use of the other ingredients in the product formulation.

The reader is advised to check local legislation for the permitted use of claims with respect to micronutrients and should note that local legislation will be subject to change.

8.6 Communication of Non-specific Health and Dietary Benefits by Food Manufacturers

As noted earlier, the formal communication of specific health and dietary benefits will be subject to local geographical guidance and in many cases, legislation. The requirements for declaring specific health and dietary claims vary and some general examples have been discussed above. Because a health or dietary claim is allowed in one geographical area it does not follow that it will be allowed elsewhere. Such variations on permitted claims most often create difficulties for the suppliers of specialist ingredients and so readers involved in product development are advised to check before or at least during the early stages of product development, the legal (or advisory) status of specialist ingredients that may be used in the product formulation and any nutrition or health claims which may be associated with them.

Consumer awareness of potential health and dietary benefits will come from many different sources; some of these are further discussed below. With a wide range of information sources available, consumer associations with the 'healthiness' of particular ingredients are quickly established. This can mean that the presence of a particular ingredient in a baked product recipe can convey an association with healthiness, even though no specific health or dietary claims are being made by the manufacturer of that product. This 'subliminal' association with healthiness is often seen where specialist ingredients are referred to as part of the product description or marketing and promotional literature. An example of such an ingredient in baking would be an oat product which contains *beta*-glucan, a material which is known to be associated with lowering cholesterol in the bloodstream and conferring other health benefits (Daou and Zhang 2012). If there are clinically proven benefits associated with the use of a particular ingredient, this may draw endorsement from medical bodies and other related reputable professional bodies as discussed below.

Other specialist ingredients with less well-substantiated nutrition and health benefits may be encountered in bakery product recipes. Often such ingredients may also be described as being 'natural' or 'unrefined' and in doing so imply that there are nutrition and health benefits by comparison with similar, though 'refined or processed' materials. Two common examples of such ingredients are flours from so-called 'ancient grains' and 'minimally-processed' sugars. Arguments for using such ingredients are often based on poorly defined and unproven studies related to their nutrition and health benefits. Frequently a common perception is that the processing or refinement of raw materials renders 'modern' food ingredients less digestible in the human gut, or in some cases deliver vaguely specified anti-nutritional characteristics. Such unspecified and medically unproven claims are largely uncharted waters for the food industry. Nevertheless some food companies do make use of these subliminal messages to convey apparent benefits associated with consuming their products by highlighting the presence of often 'trendy' ingredients on the packaging and associated marketing material. It is worth pointing out that it is a common principle in many food legislative arenas that providing health and nutrition-related information to consumers should not be done so in a misleading manner.

The concept of 'natural' ingredients and products has also become confounded with the concept of 'processed' foods; with the latter including associations with the inclusion of 'E-numbers' on product ingredients lists. In turn, this has fuelled the concept of so-called, 'clean' bakery food labels with the removal of E-numbers from the ingredient listing. The 'clean-label' concept has no legal standing, but is now widely used by specialist ingredient suppliers and has caught the imagination of the retail environment and consumers. Equally there are no clear definitions of 'natural' and 'processed' foods and this leads to significant opportunities for misconceptions and misrepresentation of research studies in popular media. Terms such 'clean-label' and 'natural' for marketing purposes should be used with great care. While they might not be prescribed in legislation, they may be construed as 'misleading' for consumers as was highlighted in a case in the UK in 2018 with respect to a complaint made to the Advertising Standards Authority (Anon 2018; Mitchell 2018a). The complaint was based on claims that a food retailer described their products as avoiding 'obscure chemicals, additives, and preservatives' and used the word 'natural' when their bread contained E-numbers. The ruling against the retailer concerned was not based on any contradiction of EU law but on the misleading nature of their marketing information.

Breadmaking is a perfect example of how 'labels' are used a means of communication. Bread is a processed food based on the manufacture of a product using wheat flour, which itself is the product of processing grain, even in the wholemeal form. The wheat used in milling is the natural product and can be seen growing in the field, everything else that follows is processed. The labelling of bread as being 'processed' in some parts of the world is associated with attempts to apply this label to the large-scale production of the fermented products in industrial-scale bakeries, as opposed to the manufacture of such products in smaller-scale, now commonly referred to as 'artisan bakeries' with (possibly) fewer ingredients. In some places products from the latter production environment are perceived to have greater, poorly specified health and nutrition benefits, and are often promoted in such a way. To date no structured medical studies have verified statements or claims that so-called artisan breads (such as those manufactured based on sour dough principles) are more digestible than other forms of bread. Only time and relevant nutritional studies will reconcile conflicting views on such topics; in the meantime consumers will continue to make their choices based on the available information, specific, or otherwise. It is somewhat ironic that the artisan and sourdough 'labels' have now migrated to products made in large-scale industrial bakeries, though in some parts of the world (e.g. northern Europe) the large-scale production of such breads has been long practised. It would appear that the artisan bread label now carries with it a marketing opportunity.

In many legislative arenas food ingredients may be permitted for use in a limited number of contexts rather that across a broad spectrum of food uses. Care should be taken to establish the precise nature of any restrictions regarding the use of a particular ingredient since attempts to implement its wider use may require legislative sanction. In some cases it is possible that the 'new' use of an already permitted food ingredient will require a submission for it use under legislative procedures which govern novel foods. A recent example in the EU (Mitchell 2018b) is based on the addition of activated charcoal to bread. Activated charcoal has a long history of being prescribed in relation to alleviation of a number of medical conditions, such as constipation, and for its potential in binding toxic materials in the digestive tract. Its recent 're-discovery', is related to its use in the manufacture of 'black bread' in Italy. While additions of vegetable carbon are permitted under EU legislation, its use was restricted to applications in fine bakery wares. In addition, health claims in the EU related to the consumption of charcoal are prescriptive and exclude its use in bread.

8.7 Communications Between Health Specialists and the Baking Industry

The relationship between nutritionists, health professionals and bakers is important but has not always been harmonious. The manufacture of bakery products is based on complex relationships between ingredients and their functionality, the ratios of ingredients to one another in the recipe and crucially, the choice of processing technology to deliver the end product (Cauvain and Young, 2006a,b). It is the ingredient–recipe–process interactions which set bakery products apart from the manufacture of many other foods. This often means that the delivery of improved nutrition via bakery products is seldom a case of simply changing the recipe or adding a new ingredient (Dewettinck et al. 2008). Issues related to the 'reformulation conundrum' for many bakery products have already been highlighted above. The reformulation of bakery products while still trying to meet consumer expectations, requires time for relevant adjustments to be made to recipes and process methods. In the kitchen at home, reducing the level of a specific ingredient in bakery products can often be readily enacted, not least because consumer expectations related to product texture are perhaps less stringent and variations in product more acceptable than would be the case in the large-scale manufacture of bakery products. It will almost certainly be the case that sensory and microbial shelf-life expectations are limited with home-based products. Differences in product qualities and consumer expectations between home-based and commercial production are not always recognised by health specialists, especially those who have limited experience or knowledge of commercial bakery practices, and this can lead to misunderstandings of the industrial feedback relevant to the development of nutritionally enhanced bakery products.

A further challenge for bakeries seeking to meet defined nutrition objectives is often associated with the use of 'replacement' ingredients; in part because so-called replacers will not have the identical functionality as the ingredient they purport to replace and in part, because the replacement materials themselves may have potential negative health connotation; some real and some perceived. The potential replacement of sodium chloride with potassium chloride represents a useful example of the dilemma that bakers often face when trying to adjust the nutrition of bakery products. The technical restrictions associated with the partial replacement of sodium chloride with the potassium salt have already been discussed. In addition to the potential technical constraints, there is the potential consumer barrier to including potassium chloride (or calcium or magnesium salts) on the product label. At the start of the initiative to reduce sodium chloride in bread in the UK, the medical value of using potassium salts was not clearly conveyed to UK bakers who subsequently opted for the gradual reduction approach, and the re-education of consumer palettes. (Increased potassium intakes are related to the reduction of cardiovascular risk factors; for example see Arburto et al. 2013.) By not using potassium chloride to partially replace sodium bakers also avoided an increase in the number of ingredients on bread product labels.

A particular problem for bakers can be the tendency for health specialist to focus on individual nutrients as has been the case with fibre, salt, fat, and most recently sugar, often with limited regard for overall product energy density. This can place bakers in the position of having satisfied one nutritional requirement at the expense of another. The ability of bakers to meet nutritional requirements while satisfying the expectation of consumers is finite. In addition to delivering 'improved' nutrition via their products, bakers may also be exhorted to limit portion sizes as part of the strategy to combat obesity. Many past nutrition studies have focused on one nutrient against one physiological effect or biomarker; this has been described by some as a 'reductionist and pharmacological approach' (Fardet 2014). The outcomes of such studies have often been contradictory and the messages for the baking industry have not always been clear. Lack of clarity with nutritional messages has led some bakers to waste significant resources in pursuing new product developments which have 'failed' as health-related messages have changed; the example of an earlier position regarding definitions and types of fats has been discussed above. It is not surprising that some bakers are reluctant to respond immediately to health specialist calls for improved nutrition, in part because of the costs involved with meeting inappropriate or failed initiatives and perhaps in part, because of a degree of scepticism as to how relevant some health messages will be at some future date. As was the case in the UK with salt reduction, most progress can be made when health specialists and bakers cooperate.

Fardet (2014) identified the need to adopt an holistic and integrative approach to food nutrition studies. He proposed that by studying the relationship between one food matrix and the physiological responses to it could form the basis for developing healthier cereal-based foods, including baked goods. In recent years the need for a 'whole systems' approach to diet and health has begun to have traction. For example, Riley et al. (2017) recognised that 'complex adaptive systems such as obesity defy [these] more linear approaches because the mass of influences continually impacts the assumptions on which the original plan was based'. These authors were contrasting a whole systems approach to diet and health with traditional programs (usually based on identifying an issue, creating a study and evaluating its outcomes) within the context of the UK's Foresight Tackling Obesities report (Butland et al. 2007) and they recognised the need to involve many partners. By involving and obtaining the support of members of baking industries, far more may be achieved in terms of beneficial impacts on consumer health and diet. Potentially this can make a greater contribution to overcoming subliminal views that foods are not medicine and reinforce the view that the nutritional enhancement of bakery foods need not result in the loss of the sensory pleasures of eating them. However, whichever approaches health specialist and bakers employ, the consumer will make the ultimate decision as to whether such dietary approaches and the products resulting from their implementation are acceptable.

8.8 Communications and Consumers

It is clear that consumers are influenced by a variety of messages; these can be from 'official' bodies through recommendations and may be linked with a particular ingredient or product. A detailed review of consumer perceptions regarding diet and health, particularly with respect to the efficacy of government and institution-led messages, is mostly outside the scope of this work. Ultimately consumer food choices do play a significant role in the healthiness of their diet and the nature of information provided to consumers with respect to health and diet cannot be completely ignored in the development of nutritionally enhanced bakery products. The food manufacturer needs to understand where their bakery products fit within current medical views and government positions on diet and health, not least so as not to mislead consumers about the 'healthiness' of their current and future products. As has been discussed above, identifying any potential nutrition claims early on in the development process is important for the delivery of new products in a cost-effective and timely manner. There are also less tangible words, phrases, and images which may be used to support the marketing of nutritionally enhanced bakery products. As has already been emphasised, labelling, and nutrition claims are usually well-regulated, but there remains the potential to use some words and phrases to imply that a product has health-related attributes; e.g. such as 'contains oats' with the subliminal link to heart health via the cholesterol lowering potential of the *beta* glucans in oats. The clear principle to follow in such contexts is that words, phrases, and images should not be used to mislead consumers regarding the healthiness of any product.

Skov and Perez-Cueto (2015) presented the results of a Danish study in which they followed the role of 'story-telling' with respect to the perceptions of bread quality. They presented students with separate samples of bread accompanied by descriptors and narratives, and asked them to rate samples on a nine-point Likert scale according to sensory variables. The first sample was presented for assessment without comment and the second with an organic or wholegrain label. With the third sample came a commentary related to the nature of the product, where it was grown and who grew it. The results showed that the more information that was given with the sample (mainly number 3), the stronger was the score for 'liking' colour and crispiness attributes; even though all of the samples presented were derived from the same product. The authors emphasised the need for food health related messages to be truthful and transparent, but at the same time concluded that the promotion of healthy eating could learn from the world of marketing and psychology. While we can learn much from such studies about the promotion of nutritionally enhanced bakery foods, manufacturers must take clear steps to deliver nutritional messages in a clear and unambiguous manner.

While it remains appropriate for bakery product manufacturers to seek to deliver new bakery products with 'stand-alone' nutritional benefits, the more recently adopted holistic view regarding diet and health should not be ignored. For example, improving the healthiness of bread for sandwich-making needs to be combined with healthier fillings. While the latter is not directly in the remit of the bakery food manufacturer, it is clear that closer collaboration with the sandwich supplier can deliver greater potential health benefits to consumers. In the UK the move to reduce salt levels in bread was initially enacted in isolation from products like sandwich fillings, so that it was possible that the overall salt level of the total product was only marginally lowered. With a more holistic approach in recent years there has been a more significant reduction in the overall salt levels in pre-packed sandwiches.

It should be remembered that all consumers are not equal; there will be variations based on regions, background, age, and just plain personal preferences for tastes and textures. Bread products are one of the most emotive topics in the food industry with many different opinions as to what are the 'right' product qualities (Cauvain 2015). In many parts of the world, health quality is now ranked equally with sensory qualities. A study of Belgian bread consumers carried out by Dewettinck et al. (2008) identified three consumer clusters; they described them as:

1) Health averse (with a strong bias to sensory attributes).
2) Health and sensory positive.
3) Sensory averse (though with no clear health preference).

This led the authors to emphasise the need for clear links between the nature of health-related information and branding in order to satisfy consumers and regulatory authorities alike. The conclusions of this particular study also re-emphasised the key role that sensory qualities play in consumer acceptance of bakery products; for some consumers this appears to be at the expense of healthiness.

8.9 Media Communicated Information and Disinformation

The traditional forms of media, such as print, film, radio, and television, have all been used to communicate with consumers on matters of diet and health, often with information provided by governments and other associated bodies. In recent years the rise of the internet and social media have become more popular means of obtaining advice on diet and health. Government and other related bodies have recognised the value of using the internet to communicate information on health and diet and readily provide advice on-line, via mobile apps and through social media channels, such as blogs and Twitter (Zhou et al. 2018). A study published in 2013 (Lee 2013) found that around 72% of adults in the USA had searched for health-related information in the previous 12-month period, demonstrating the potential power (and risks) of being able to access on-line information. Government and other related bodies providing nutritional information commonly do so by providing down-loadable documents, in many ways the equivalent of the traditional printed booklet. Such documents provide a greater level of detail beyond the headlines and summary paragraphs which commonly greet on-line users when they engage in on-line searches. It is important therefore that key messages are quickly and readily conveyed to the searcher, both to satisfy their immediate needs and to identify the availability and value of more relevant detailed documents.

The advent of the internet and social media has significantly increased the availability to health-related information for consumers. However, increased availability does not necessarily increase the 'value' of such information, not least because almost anyone can post health-related information on a web page, blog, or comment through social media. The speed at which information can be exchanged using social media means that messages can cover the globe in a matter of a few minutes; in the modern vernacular a single post can 'go viral'. All too often viral posts tend to be negative in tone and often lack validity. This can be a problem with respect to dietary information, especially that which is initially posted by individuals who have a large number of followers. This has given rise to the phenomena of the 'celebrity diet' and is fuelled by the appetite of many consumers for information in 'small bites' and simple solutions to their (complex) dietary needs. A similar problem exists with nutritional and dietary information made available through more traditional media such as print, not least because journalists writing for more popular papers and magazines commonly re-hash outdated information or only access the abstracts of current nutrition research.

The advent of modern methods of communication does place a greater emphasis on nutritionists and food manufacturers to exchange information more effectively. For the food manufacturer it is important that nutrition-related information presented to them is clear and unequivocal so they have clear goals for developing nutritionally enhanced bakery products. This requires that clear distinctions are made between research studies and more widely accepted nutritional guidelines and recommendations relevant to consumers, not least so that the manufacturer can engage in informed debate with their customers. It is worth remembering that the latter will not always be the consumer but is increasingly it has become the food retailer.

For the bakery food manufacturer there is an increasing need to understand advances and trends in the field of human nutrition so they can more readily choose appropriate raw materials and develop new products. Equally it is incumbent on the manufacturer to ensure that all dietary information on their products is clear and meets the relevant regulatory requirements. Much product information can be accessed by consumers using the internet, even before a product is purchased and while social media has advantages for promoting bakery products, especially newly-developed ones, it is important that marketing messages do not mislead consumers with respect to the nutritional value and healthiness of bakery products.

8.10 Conclusions

The need for presenting clear and unequivocal information on the healthiness and nutritional value of bakery products to consumers is self-evident. The vast majority of bakery foods are the subject of regulations designed to ensure that such objectives are achieved. Though the precise form in which composition and nutrition data may take will vary on a regional basis, the main areas related to macro- and micronutrient claims and composition are essentially common. As well as ensuring that the statutory requirements are met, bakery food manufacturers need to ensure that any supplementary information presented does not mislead on the healthiness of bakery products.

There have been significant changes in the manner in which information is communicated to consumers on health and diet. The advent of the internet and the rise of mass communication through social media, have brought both opportunities and risks for food manufacturers. Individuals can now readily access a significant level of detail with respect to health and diet, though not all of the available information comes from verifiable sources and the potential for the spread of disinformation is significant. Nutritionists, researchers, and bakers all have significant roles to play in making good quality information available; a process which starts with good communication amongst themselves if sustainable nutrition enhancement of bakery products and positive contributions to consumer diet and health are to be achieved.

References

Anon. (2018) Pret rapped over 'natural' food claim. *British Baker*, May, 4.

Arburto, N.J., Hanson, S., Gutierrez, H. et al. (2013). Effect of increased potassium intake on cardiovascular risk factors and disease: systematic review and meta-analyses. *British Medical Journal* 346: f1378. https://doi.org/10.1136/bmj.f1378.

Butland, B., Jebb, S., Kopelman, P. et al. (2007). *Foresight: Tackling Obesities: Future Voices – Project Report*, 2e. London, UK: Department of Innovation, Universities and Skills, HMSO.

Carlisle, S. and Hanlon, P. (2014). Connecting food, well-being and environmental sustainability. *Critical Public Health* 24 (4): 405–417.

Cauvain, S.P. (2003). Bread industry and consumer expectations regarding organic bakery products in the European Union. (In German. *Getreide, Mehl & Brot* 57: 100–107.

Cauvain, S.P. (2015). *Technology of Breadmaking*, 3e. Berlin: Springer International Publishing.

Cauvain, S.P. and Young, L.S. (2006a). *Bakery Products; Science, Technology and Practice*. Oxford, UK: Blackwell.

Cauvain, S.P. and Young, L.S. (2006b). *The Chorleywood Bread Process*. Cambridge, UK: Woodhead Publishing.

Daou, C. and Zhang, H. (2012). Oat beta-glucan: its role in health promotion and prevention of diseases. *Comprehensive Reviews in Food Science and Safety* 11: 355–365.

Devaney, B.L. and Barr, S.I. (2002). DRI, EAR, RDA, AI, UL; Making sense of this alphabet soup. *Nutrition Today* 37 (6): 226–232.

Dewettinck, K., Van Bockstacle, F., Kuhne, B. et al. (2008). Nutritional value of bread: influence of processing, food interaction and consumer preference. *Journal of Cereal Science* 48: 243–257.

Fardet, A. (2014). New approaches to studying the potential health benefits of cereals: from reductionism to holism. *Cereal Foods World* 59 (5): 224–229.

Hegarty, V. (1992). *Nutrition: Food and the Environment*. St. Paul, MN: Eagan Press.

Jackson, M., Harrison, P., Swinburn, B., and Lawrence, M. (2014). Unhealthy food, integrated marketing communication and power: a critical analysis. *Critical Public Health* 24 (4): 489–505.

Lee, R. (2013) E-patients and their hunt for health information. *Scientific Report*, Pew Research Centre, Washington, DC. www.pewinternet.org/2013/10/10/e-patients-and-their-hunt-for-health-information/

Mitchell, J. (2018a) Defining natural. *British Baker,* June, 15.

Mitchell, J. (2018b) Not such a grey area. *British Baker,* April, 15.

Prasad, K.N. (2011). *Micronutrients in Health and Disease*. Boca Raton, FL: CRC Press.

Riley, J., Saunders, J., and Blackshaw, J. (2017). Whole systems obesity programme. *Perspectives in Public Health* 137 (3): 146–147.

Skov, L.R. and Perez-Cueto, A. (2015). How storytelling can bias sensory perceptions among young students. *Perspectives in Public Health* 135 (4): 174–175.

Zhou, J., Liu, F., and Zhou, H. (2018). Understanding health food messages on Twitter for health literacy promotion. *Perspectives in Public Health* 138 (3): 173–179.

Glossary

While there is a degree of commonality associated with the terminology used in the manufacture of bakery products, there are regional variations; this glossary is provided to help readers who are less familiar with some of the baking terms used in this work.

ascorbic acid The common chemical name for vitamin C. It is used as a flour and dough modification agent. Sometimes referred to as an 'oxidant'. It is chemically a reducing agent, but is converted during dough mixing to dehydroascorbic acid in the presence of atmospheric oxygen and the ascorbic acid oxidase enzyme in the flour. In this converted form it acts as the oxidising agent.

asparagines A non-essential amino acid nutritionally involved in the formation of acrylamide in foods.

bakers' yeast The microorganism which ferments sugars to produce carbon dioxide and alcohol.

baking powder A mixture of a food grade acid and a bicarbonate source which delivers carbon dioxide gas. In double–acting baking powders two different acids are used to control the rate of carbon dioxide release during processing and baking.

barley Cereal commonly used to produce malt extract and extract. May be found in speciality bakery products.

biscuits and cookies Thin, baked confectionery products based on flour, sugar, and fat, with a low moisture content (typically less than 5%) and hard or crumbly textures.

bread improver (dough conditioner) Individual or mixtures of functional ingredients added during breadmaking to 'improve' the processing of the dough or the qualities of the final product.

Baking Technology and Nutrition: Towards a Healthier World, First Edition.
Stanley P. Cauvain and Rosie H. Clark.

cake Item of flour confectionery. Typically, recipes contain fat (oil) and sugar. The products have a light, aerated texture and baked moisture content in the region 20–25%. Sponge cakes are lower in recipe oil or fat.

Chorleywood Bread Process A breadmaking process developed in the UK in which all the ingredients are mixed together in one single operation to a fixed energy (work input). The mixed and developed dough is transferred directly to the divider with no resting period.

coalescence The process by which two or more individual gas bubbles fuse to become one larger one.

dietary fibre The edible parts plants which are resistant to digestion and absorption in the human small intestine, with complete or partial fermentation in the large intestine. Dietary fibre components typically include; polysaccharides, (e.g. cellulose, hemicellulose), oligosaccharides (short-chain polysaccharides), and complex carbohydrates, such as resistant starch.

dough development and gas retention The modification of the properties of gluten in a wheat flour dough (mainly through mixing and kneading) so that it has the appropriate rheological and gas retention properties which will enable it to deliver the appropriate final product quality.

dough rheology The term which describes the collective behavioural properties of dough when it is placed under the stresses and strains of processing. Wheat flour doughs are described as visco-elastic; i.e. having viscous and elastic properties. Elasticity is a property of materials which allows then to regain their shape after any deforming force has been removed. In baking contexts, the extensibility of the gluten network is an important rheological property.

emulsifiers Substances which are soluble in fat and water. Used in bakery products to form stable emulsions and improve product quality (volume and softness). Commonly used emulsifiers include:

- *DATA esters (DATEM).* Mainly used in the manufacture of bread and fermented products. Confers stability and strength to dough.
- *Monoglyceride (glycerol mono-stearate).* Used for its ability to incorporate air during cake batter mixing and as anti-staling agent in breadmaking.
- *SSL (Sodium steroyld-2-lactylate).* Used to confer stability of bread and fermented doughs.

enzymes Biological catalysts with specific functions. They are commonly used in bread and cake improvers. Those enzymes of greater interest in baking include:

- *Amylases.* Generic description applied to the enzyme combination – *alpha* and *beta* – which breaks down starch in wheat flour to yield maltose sugar.
- Cereal *alpha*-amylase which occurs naturally in wheat and barley flours.
- Liquid malt extract and malt flour prepared from malted barley (or wheat).
- *Maltase.* Which breaks down the disaccharide maltose and supports fermentation by bakers' yeast.
- *Glucose oxidase.* Which oxidises glucose to gluconic acid and forms hydrogen peroxide, which is considered to contribute to dough oxidation.
- *Lipases.* Which react with fats (triglycerides) and break them down.
- *Protease (proteinase).* Which breaks down proteins.

epithelial layer/tissue The layer in the human body through which all materials entering or leaving must ultimately cross. Epithelial layers protect underlying tissues.

equilibrium relative humidity (ERH)/water activity (a_w) That unique humidity at which moisture is neither lost from nor gained by a baked product, expressed as a percentage. In a product wrapped in an impermeable film, the ERH will indicate that the rate of moisture evaporation from the product equals the rate of moisture condensation onto the product. Water activity is the ratio of the vapour pressure in a bakery product (p) to that of pure water (p_o); thus $a_w = p/p_o$ at equilibrium for a given temperature. At equilibrium conditions and a given temperature, $a_w = ERH/100$.

fat and oils Edible triglycerides of different origins. Plant oils are most commonly used in baking. The terms are often used to distinguish between a product which is liquid (oil) or solid (fat) at temperatures around 20°C. Key properties in baking include:

- *Melting point.* Indicates the temperature at which a fat becomes an oil.
- *NMR value.* The proportion of a fat which is solid at a given temperature.

- *Slip point.* The temperature at which a solid fat turns to oil. Named after the method used to determine the relevant temperature.
- *Solid fat content (SFC) or Solid fat index (SFI).* The proportion of a composite fat which is solid at a given temperature.

fermentation Process by which bakers' yeast acting on dough sugars and produces carbon dioxide gas. Commonly linked with the resting of the bulk dough for a fixed period of time after mixing and before dividing. Fermentation also occurs in the prover but as this associated with individual dough pieces, bakers tend to use the term proof. There is a brief period of fermentation in the oven before bakers' yeast is inactivated by heat.

first (intermediate) proof A short period of time between the moulding steps applied to dough pieces, to modify dough rheology (allows the dough to 'relax'). Carried out in an intermediate or 'overhead' prover.

foam to sponge conversion In baking, the transition from a matrix in which gas bubbles are held separately (foam) to the one which has an open and inter-connected cellular structure (sponge). Examples are dough to bread and batter to cake crumb.

furans Organic compounds formed during thermal processing.

gluten The matrix which forms in wheat flour dough when the hydrated proteins gliadin (the main allergic component in coeliac disease) and glutenin proteins are subjected to the input of energy from mixing and kneading.

gluten-free Ingredients or products which do not contain gluten-forming proteins.

hydration The addition of water to a substance or material and the process by which wheat proteins, starch, and fibres absorb water during breadmaking.

hygroscopic Materials which readily absorb water (e.g. salt and sugar) are said to be hygroscopic.

laminated products A sub-group of bakery products based on the creation of interleaved layers of fat and dough. Examples include:

- *Crackers.* A thin, flaky textured product, with a moisture content of less than 5%. May contain yeast.
- *Croissant.* A yeasted product cylindrical or crescent-shaped.
- *Danish pastry.* Rich dough formulae, commonly yeasted.
- *Puff pastry.* Un-yeasted, laminated product.The folding process used to build up individual fat and dough layers is known as lamination.

mixing (and kneading) The bringing together of separate ingredients to form an homogeneous mass. The transfer of energy in bread dough may also be referred to as kneading.

moulding The process by which individual dough pieces are manipulated to the required final shape before proving.

no-time dough A dough making process in which the there is no significant delay in transferring the dough from the mixer to the divider.

proteins Polymers of many hundreds of amino acids composed of carbon, hydrogen, oxygen, and nitrogen (sometimes with sulphur and phosphorous).

proving (proof, proofing) The final fermentation stage which occurs within individual dough pieces before transfer to the oven. Carried out under controlled temperatures and humidity-controlled conditions in a prover. During proof the dough pieces expand, and the gluten network relaxes becoming more extensible.

reducing agents Ingredients which are used to modify dough rheology in baking e.g. inactivated yeast, L-cysteine hydrochloride and sodium metabisulphite.

rotary moulder Equipment used in the shaping of biscuit and cookie dough pieces. The dough being pressed into a pre-cut mould on rotating cylinder.

rye Cereal used in the manufacture of bread. The flour lacks the strength of wheat gluten and is dark in colour. Often used in sour dough manufacture. May be mixed with wheat flour.

salt Term commonly applied to sodium chloride – common salt. Residual salts result from chemical reactions of an acid with an alkali in baking powders.

sheeting The action of passing dough or paste between pairs of parallel rollers to gradually reduce its thickness.

shortcrust pastry Savoury or sweetened paste used for the manufacture of meat (savoury) or fruit pies (sweetened).

sour dough Method of producing bread based on fermentation and acid formation from a combination of naturally occurring lactic acid bacteria (in flour) and wild yeasts.

sponge and dough breadmaking process A breadmaking process in which a portion of the ingredients are made into a separate dough (the sponge) and fermented for a period before being mixed with the remaining ingredients to make the final dough. Sponge fermentation times may vary from 1–18 h according and the proportion of the flour used 10–60%.

starch A plant carbohydrate which is a polymer of glucose. Found in the endosperm of grains and different plants. There are two important forms with different properties; amylose (straight chain) and amylopectin (branched chain). The breakdown of starch by amylase enzymes supports fermentation during breadmaking. During baking, starch changes from a crystalline (ordered) to an amorphous (i.e. unorganised) structure after hydration and under the influence of heat in the oven. The gelatinisation temperature is important in determining final product quality. In a baked loaf, retrogradation of starch is a key to the staling mechanism in which bread crumb firms without losing moisture.

sugar(s) Compounds of carbon, hydrogen, and oxygen which may contain 3–7 carbon atoms defined by the molecular formula $C_nH_{2n}O_n$. In common parlance, sugar is most closely associated with sucrose (a disaccharide comprising glucose and fructose). Other sugars commonly encountered in baking include:

- *Fructose.* A 6-carbon sugar found in fruits and honey. 1.7 times sweeter than sucrose. Also known as laevulose.
- *Glucose.* A 6-carbon chain monosaccharide, also known as dextrose. Often used in the syrup form. Present in the human blood stream as the result of the metabolic breakdown of foods.
- *Maltose.* A disaccharide broken down by the enzyme maltase associated with bakers' yeast to yield carbon dioxide gas and alcohol during dough fermentation.

wheat The major cereal used to yield flour for the manufacture of bakery products. Composed of branny materials (13%), embryo (sometimes called germ) (2%), and starchy endosperm (85%). The protein contents and qualities vary according to the variety, agronomic practices and geographical location in which wheat is grown. Wholemeal wheat flour is 100% of the wheat grain ground to flour between stones or steel rollers. White flour commonly refers to the starchy endosperm separated from the bran and germ during milling. There are different grades of white flour with varying properties.

Index

Baking Technology and Nutrition: Towards a Healthier World, First Edition.
Stanley P. Cauvain and Rosie H. Clark.

Printed and bound by CPI Group (UK) Ltd, Croydon, CR0 4YY

17/09/2026

14004203 0001